Pharma's Prescription

How the Right Technology can Save the Pharmaceutical Business

Pharma's Prescription

How the Right Technology can Save the Pharmaceutical Business

Kamal Biswas
Partner, Global Life Sciences Consulting
Infosys Limited

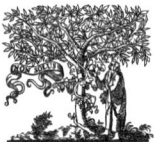

AMSTERDAM • BOSTON • HEIDELBERG • LONDON
NEW YORK • OXFORD • PARIS • SAN DIEGO
SAN FRANCISCO • SINGAPORE • SYDNEY • TOKYO

Academic Press is an imprint of Elsevier

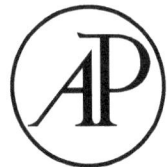

Academic Press is an imprint of Elsevier
32 Jamestown Road, London NW1 7BY, UK
225 Wyman Street, Waltham, MA 02451, USA
525 B Street, Suite 1800, San Diego, CA 92101-4495, USA

Notice
No responsibility is assumed by the publisher for any injury and/or damage to persons
or property as a matter of products liability, negligence or otherwise, or from any use
or operation of any methods, products, instructions or ideas contained in the material
herein. Because of rapid advances in the medical sciences, in particular, independent
verification of diagnoses and drug dosages should be made

British Library Cataloguing-in-Publication Data
A catalogue record for this book is available from the British Library

Library of Congress Cataloging-in-Publication Data
A catalog record for this book is available from the Library of Congress

ISBN: 978-0-12-407662-4

For information on all Academic Press publications
visit our website at www.store.elsevier.com

Typeset by TNQ Books and Journals

Transferred to Digital Printing in 2014

Contents

Foreword

Any book on the pharmaceutical industry is critical to the success of its professionals. This book is one such and its arrival is not a moment too soon! This industry has created wonders in the past by developing life-saving drugs. The pharmaceutical companies have helped extend our life expectancy to a level beyond our imagination. We are a much healthier society today with less everyday health issues to worry about, thanks to the pharmaceutical industry.

However, the use of technology to drive business improvement in the pharmaceutical industry is still in its infancy. When we started the Life Sciences practice at Infosys over a decade ago, our intention was to help enhance the industry's innovation engine by using modern technologies and solutions that have helped other industries. Computer-based drug design, virtual clinical trials, drug dosage modeling, 3D printing of human tissues and organs and patient monitoring and support in real-time have already made the industry much more innovative than before. Several technology solutions have streamlined manufacturing operations to reduce the cost of production to make drugs more affordable. We have helped several of the top pharmaceutical companies to drive innovations and reduce costs. Today, we help them with the effective use of digital and mobile technologies to create closer links with the patients and physicians. We help track the movement of medicines from the manufacturing shop floor to the patients' cabinets using technologies to reduce counterfeit drugs.

Kamal is one of the founding members of the Infosys Life Sciences practice and has led our journey of a technology-driven pharmaceutical business transformation. Kamal's inquiring mind has taken him to various business functions in the pharmaceutical industry. He has gained insights from drug development labs, has worked in manufacturing plants, and has introduced new products in several countries before moving to consulting in the management and technology world. With close to two decades of industry work and consulting experience in the US, Europe and Asia with several global pharmaceutical companies, his ideas resonate well with the needs of the industry. Kamal's book is the culmination of his life's work and reads like a professional diary of a pharmaceutical industry insider.

Kamal is highly appreciated for his client-centric approach in solving business problems. This has made him a trusted advisor to many pharmaceutical companies across the globe. He is also a people leader. His customer-centric approach and people leadership qualities are reflected in his book as well. He insists that every individual in the industry should always think about how the next person in the chain would use his or her output. Kamal believes that the ultimate index of satisfaction of our work is measured by how much of a smile we bring to the faces of our customers.

The book reflects Kamal's expertise and experience in strengthening the pharmaceutical business and technology interface. He has described the business processes of the entire pharmaceutical value chain for easy understanding for newbies to the industry and the technologists. He has also explained the technology basics for business stakeholders to prepare them for making better decisions in using technology to improve their business.

Kamal highlights the need for making medicines more accessible and affordable to people across the globe. He believes rightly that the role of IT in making this dream a reality is significant. For this, Kamal exhorts pharmaceutical business executives to embrace technology wholeheartedly and accept new ways of working. As an FDA-certified pharmaceutical manufacturing professional and ISO9000 quality auditor, Kamal draws attention to the greater need for transparency in quality and compliance as the industry moves towards generics and business shifts into the emerging markets.

This book is a practitioner's diary. Kamal has cited several industry examples to explain his thought leadership. He has described top pharmaceutical industry turnaround stories that will help improve the industry operations globally and bring in innovative and preventive therapies.

I admire Kamal's passionate work in the Life Sciences industry. Such passion keeps him motivated to work hard, and smart. It inspires others in the industry to innovate with a sense of altruism. I wish him great success!

Narayana Murthy
Chairman Emeritus – Infosys Limited, Bangalore, India

Acknowledgements

Firstly, I would like to show my respect and convey my deepest gratitude to Mr. Narayana Murthy for writing the foreword. I wrote the book but it got life with Mr. Murthy's touch. I don't have the words to show my appreciation to him for taking time out of his extremely busy schedule. My sincere thanks to this visionary leader for making my dream come true. I also thank Mr. Pandu for his support in putting this into Mr. Murthy's schedule and making it happen.

I am deeply grateful for the constant encouragement and motivation given to me by several people: Jith, the global Head of Infosys Life Sciences practice; Sandeep Raju, the charismatic leader who brought me to the world of technology-driven business transformation; Kristine Jones, the leader from Elsevier Inc.; Noushir Jagmag, Infosys marketing leader; Anuj Kumar, the Life Sciences delivery leader; Ashu Tandon, the pharmaceutical sales leader with whom I started my Life Sciences journey at Infosys; and my wife, Koyel, for resolutely encouraging me to take the leap. Without them spurring me on, I would still have been thinking of this as just one more project.

This book would not have been possible without the active support from some of the chapter co-authors and reviewers. Jeremy Pincus of GSK; Kevin Nicolas, Gurdeep S. Rooprai and Sandeep Kumar from Infosys; Scott Owen Mason of Novartis and Lu Ann Binda from Pfizer. They all played a large role in crafting business problems, debating problem statements and helping to design technology-driven solutions to improve the pharmaceutical industry.

I could not have completed this book without strong support from the Infosys Life Sciences consulting team. While the whole team has shown not only a huge sense of excitement, many of them became actively involved. I would like to express my gratitude to Dr. Nandini Diwakar; Amutha Devi, PhD; Ankasha Tejam, PhD; Sumehra Patterson, Kirti Jindal, Shreela Murugesan, Anuradha Roy and Himanshu Parmar. They are all experts in various aspects of pharmaceutical business and have spent several hours providing input, critique content and support with the additional information needed.

My sincere thanks to the Infosys team in management consulting, business technology services and client services groups with whom

I got the opportunity to work with and gain knowledge from to create this practitioner's diary. Raj Joshi, Rajesh Murthy, Mind Tsai, Subhro Mallik, Ashish Goel, Ashish Jandial, to name a few, who have helped gain significant knowledge from various industries. I would not have gathered the expertise and experience required to write this book without the support from my colleagues and friends. Thank you all.

I want to thank many of my industry friends, clients and ex-colleagues from Pfizer, Novartis, GSK, BMS, Merck, Johnson & Johnson, AstraZeneca and Abbott, McKinsey, Accenture, Booz, Cap Gemini, Cognizant, Deloitte, PwC, TCS, Wipro, HCL, SAP, Oracle, Apple and Google. They have all enriched my knowledge of industry and technology that will help the pharmaceutical industry move to the next level.

Heartfelt thanks to my publishing team from Elsevier Inc., including Kristine Jones, Andy Albrecht, Matt Limbert, Marieke O'Connor, Julia Haynes, Ofelia Chernock, Shannon Stanton, Soo Hamilton and others for their ongoing support with the book during the development, design, copy-editing, production and marketing phases.

I would like to thank the Infosys research team led by Nasir for supporting my hypotheses with meaningful data and information. The research team has also identified more hypotheses to make the book more interesting. It would not have been possible to get the book to this stage without support from Infosys Labs—SVS and his team for helping me with all the steps in the publication process; and Sarma, Anindya Sircar from IP cell to ensure compliance. My sincere thanks to Jay Akasie for his excellent review and feedback.

I had to write this book without impacting on my day job, which at times is very demanding. I had to take the authoring work home. My family time has suffered for several months—every evening and weekend—and I had to skip baseball practice and games with my son over and over again. This book would not have been possible at all without the support, courage and the taking on of additional family responsibilities by my wife, Koyel and our son, Rudro. I love you both for helping me out with the completion of this milestone.

Support and courage came from many friends and family from around the world. Thank you all for your encouragement.

Kamal Biswas
Partner, Global Life Sciences Consulting
Edison, New Jersey, USA

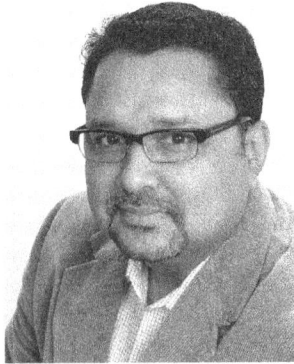

Kamal Biswas is a Partner and Leader of the Global Life Sciences Consulting Practice at Infosys. He has nearly two decades of hands-on experience in the pharmaceutical industry. He worked for 10 years in pharmaceutical manufacturing operations, technical R&D, and new product launches.

Kamal moved into management consulting to drive forward industry growth and margin preservation, accelerate innovation and improve compliance. He has worked with many pharmaceutical majors including Ciba Geigy, Novartis, Pfizer, GSK, Aventis, J&J and BMS, either as an employee or as a consultant. He has developed several technology-driven solutions that have helped pharmaceutical companies transform business functions to enhance business values for the company and customers.

Kamal has worked in Europe, Asia and the Americas, and currently lives with his family in the US. He has a Masters in Engineering & Technology, went to business school for International Marketing, is a certified ISO9000 Quality Auditor, and is a member of the board in several industry forums. Kamal is a strategist and evangelist of pharmaceutical business transformation through non-traditional methods and frequently speaks at industry councils.

When Stephanie was born in Monaco in 2012 she was born with a 90-year life expectancy; once this level of life expectancy becomes a reality all over the world the pharmaceutical industry will have kept its promise. With the advancement in technology this could be a viable reality and could improve even more in the near future. Human life expectancy has more than doubled in the last century and we are now moving towards tripling it soon. Access to clean drinking water made the initial impact, but the advent of pharmaceutical products has extended it considerably more.

When Linda first finds a lump in her left breast at the age of 39, she is very worried. She is first comforted and placated by her physician for several reasons—firstly, it looks noncancerous and secondly science and technology have advanced enough to find a cure with a higher success rate. The doctor's first prediction is incorrect and Linda's lump proves to be cancerous, but the prognosis is still good. With the advancement of genetic engineering and technology today, scientists have identified several gene subtypes, each with a unique genetic fingerprint to diagnose breast cancer with a survival rate of over 90%. This was less than 50% two decades ago.

In Liberia or Sierra Leone over 40% of people have been a victim of counterfeit drugs. Counterfeit medicine—a deliberately mislabeled drug with respect to identity or source—is a huge problem in sub-Saharan Africa and it needs to be stopped. Sproxil, the social enterprise to empower consumers, uses cell phones to text a code on any medication they have, to see if it's counterfeit. With only 4% of households in Africa having internet connectivity, a cell phone-based solution is trying to crack down on counterfeit medicine issues. This and other similar mobile technology solutions can easily combat the USD 600 billion counterfeit industry [1a].

Today, half of the world's population lives on less than two dollars a day and a billion on less than one dollar a day. The advancement of healthcare and technology has to be far more affordable than it is today. So, the task isn't just to find innovative ways to treat but also at an affordable cost.

Christina's appeal on a website says it all. Her 35-year-old husband and father of their two children is suffering from Primary Sclerosing Cholangitis (PSC), a chronic liver disease, and the only recovery option is to do a liver transplant. He has been on the waiting list for over a year and has almost lost hope in finding a donor before he breathes his last. A liver recipient currently waits between seven months and four years and almost one out of four of them die before a donor is found.

Christina doesn't yet know how she will raise money for the transplant. A liver transplant can typically cost up to half-a-million US dollars. This is not affordable for this single earner family of four. But Christina's situation will change soon with the help of a 3D liver printing solution. Organovo has printed functional human liver tissue— yes, liver tissue which will produce a fully functional liver as 3D printing matures further [1b]. This will eliminate the long waiting list and make transplants affordable to all. Technology will make this miracle work.

The pharmaceutical industry has brought significant changes to our lives in two waves: firstly by inventing medicines that cure disease and secondly by inventing newer and more efficient techniques with higher success. Technology plays a colossal role in improving healthcare in society today.

However, things are not as shiny as they look. The majority of the world's population does not have access to medicines. Although individuals as well as most governments see health as a priority and access to health as a right, 80% of the world's population have no or very little access to medicine. Business and technology combined have a huge task to accomplish—make medicine accessible to most of the world's population. The pharmaceutical business is central in making this happen throughout the world's healthcare ecosystem, along with providers and payers and with the help of innovative technologies. The industry has done a terrific job in improving medicines—they have very successfully brought in several new medicines and there are brilliant people around to make pharmaceutical science more meaningful to society. On the other hand, technology is constantly changing with newer and better solutions to serve human health. Although both business and technology teams have done extremely well in their own fields, there's a great opportunity to combine the two for a much better result. This can happen through focusing more on the interface between business and Information Technology (IT). Business needs better understanding of IT possibilities to improve business outcomes and IT needs to understand business functions and challenges better to apply newer technologies more meaningfully. This book entirely focuses on this interface.

In mid-2000, I led a team to build an IT solution for analyzing existing product mechanism of action and predicting the possibilities of re-purposing them for other disease conditions at one of the top five global pharmaceutical companies in the US. On one occasion, when an R&D scientist was explaining the business process, he used the term "GxP" and an analyst in my team asked him, "What is GxP?" The scientist paused for several seconds before carrying on. He saw this as a very silly question as he expected anyone who works in this area to be well versed with the foundational industry regulations, e.g. Good x Practice (GxP). It was, however, a valid question from the analyst as this was her first project in a pharmaceutical company. Though both of them were correct in their thinking, and even if we believe that no question is entirely wrong or irrelevant as it always removes ambiguity from the mind of the inquirer, it doesn't always offer value to everyone. This reminded me of the story of the middle school student who had to find "X" in a triangle. The student had circled the "X" and written "Here it is". This story makes everyone laugh, but the student was logical—he found the "X" in the diagram as if he was playing a treasure hunt game and wasn't sitting for the math exam. The examiner did of course expect a different level of maturity for better acceptance. These stories reflect the need for stronger basic knowledge in the area of work for higher success. The IT team needs to know the fundamental elements of pharmaceutics and business should have a basic understanding of technology for harmonious teamwork.

Today, everyone in the business needs to be a team player. Individual excellence needs to be expanded to form part of the goals of the larger team to make a business successful. An effective team can be created only if one understands what others want from you or how your output can offer and add value to others. Knowing what others do and using your deliverables is not easy. When I worked as a process design engineer in a pharmaceutical R&D laboratory, I always wondered how a lab-scale process is converted to mass-scale production. This question took me to the product scale-up lab, then to manufacturing plant design work and finally to the shop-floor production operations. I couldn't stop there; my next question was "How is the product I manufacture sold in the market" and that led me to the product launch team. My desire to always understand the next step of what I do led me to work across various functions. When I moved to the manufacturing shop floor operation from the scale-up team, I wondered if my earlier job would not have been more meaningful if I had known more about the production operation. Knowing the customer is the best way to improve your own work. This brought me to the realization that every executive, manager, supervisor or technician in the ecosystem should build on this desire to understand how their services are used by their customers.

However, moving between job functions is easier said than done. Hence, I wanted to write this book to provide a quick overview of all the business areas without actually having to work in those areas. This book will allow the entire community to quickly understand various functions in the pharmaceutical value chain well enough to make their own work more meaningful. A wider view of the industry will help readers become aware of their internal and external customers and it will make their daily work more customer-centric.

As the pharmaceutical industry goes through a series of challenges including declining topline growth, a dried product pipeline, increasing regulatory demands and changing customer needs, the role of technology increases remarkably. Every company is being challenged by shareholders to justify high R&D investments while earnings per share are shrinking every year. The industry response includes restructuring of business organizations to make them nimble, increasing the focus on customers, identifying non-core work to be executed through external partners and using innovative technologies to make operations more simple, efficient and productive.

Pharma's Prescription is meant to prepare stakeholders of the pharmaceutical business and technology interface to take on the journey of technology-driven business improvements together. When I moved into the IT consulting world, I found it difficult to have meaningful business conversations with people who had limited business knowledge in spite of having vast technical knowledge. This knowledge gap prevents pharmaceutical and technology companies from effectively applying the right technologies which will improve business operations. Technology companies fail to proactively identify more complex industry problems due to lack of business knowledge, and pharmaceutical business stakeholders are unable to secure the technological benefits due to a limited understanding of available IT solutions. This book will help business executives, IT executives, analysts and programmers to understand the pharmaceutical business process across the entire value chain as well as IT solutions that can improve business outcomes. These business and IT leaders will significantly enhance their preparedness for and understanding of technology innovations, the potential impact on the pharmaceutical industry and within their business function. Readers will be able to use the knowledge to discuss strategic and operational initiatives, both with their business and IT stakeholders.

Pharma's Prescription includes several existing and emerging challenges and capabilities the industry will need in order to remain profitable in the business and continue improving healthcare. This includes redesigning the pharmaceutical business model to improve R&D output through crowd sourcing or preparing more effectively for complex global regulatory requirements. Examples are given of how technology solutions can be used to solve business problems and bring in additional business capabilities. Business and IT readers will appreciate these examples and learn how to apply them in their work areas by setting tangible goals rather than having unrealistic aspirations.

There is a need for a change in leadership mindset as well. While the pharmaceutical industry spends the highest amount of all the industries on R&D, their IT investment is not comparable to some of the leading industries. This contradiction needs to be reduced to save the pharmaceutical business. Pharmaceutical industry needs an IT shot in the arm—and not a moment too soon. The executive suite is mired in a bygone era, a time when large, well-funded pharmaceutical R&D produced blockbuster drugs. Today, the pharmaceutical business needs to change substantially in order to save itself and avoid a crisis.

Chapter 1

Pharma Health—Critical Parts Need Redesigning

Once again, Randy wakes up with severe knee pain but has to get ready for work. His manager, the company's CFO, needs him to prepare for the quarterly announcement. Randy is in such pain that he can't even move, but he's not that worried. Current treatment options using advanced technologies have made his treatment simple and easy. Randy takes his smartphone, opens the "gene" application and attaches a "blood test unit" through the tiny USB port. The "gene" application does everything from there. It takes a blood sample for gene-sequencing. The sequencing is done in a few seconds and it matches against a standard pattern to identify the problem. The system automatically compares the problem with the treatment options and presents two treatment options to Randy on his smartphone. Option 1 is to temporarily block the pain signal to the brain so that he is not bothered by pain. Option 2 is to consult a physician immediately to discuss a long-term solution. Randy chooses the first option as he can't skip going to the office today. The "gene" application then prepares the symptom and therapy option mapping and sends it to a physician for approval. One of the online physicians approves the therapy. The application gives Randy two options for the medication—he can pick it up from any chemist/drugstore on his way to the office or he can engage his 3D printer to print it at home. The time from diagnosis to cure takes just 30 minutes.

Randy's "gene" application isn't available yet but neither is a science fiction. The healthcare industry will make this application available in the next few years. And when it becomes available, it will open up a whole new world—treatment options, medicine selection and delivery, physician consultation, reimbursement, etc. These new ways of working will ask for a redesign of several stakeholders in the healthcare ecosystem including the pharmaceutical business. The fast advancement of technology may make this available very soon; however, the regulators need to

Pharma's Prescription. http://dx.doi.org/10.1016/B978-0-12-407662-4.00001-5

accept this transformational treatment possibility. When it becomes reality, this will be the best use of the human genome project outcomes.

The view of the patient today is: "When it comes to my health I don't care how much it costs". The government, on the other hand, insists: "The entire healthcare industry is inflated, everyone needs to focus on reducing cost". But the payer says: "I won't pay the manufacturer if their product is ineffective". So, what would the pharmaceutical industry do in this changed scenario? The pharmaceutical industry isn't part of the core healthcare ecosystem along with the other stakeholders—physician, provider, payer and patients. They have always been seen as having monetary gain as their first priority and are kept outside of the ecosystem. The industry has to prove its willingness and ability to improve healthcare and demonstrate that they are not just there to make money. This means a better connection with patients, extending services to go beyond selling medicines, and focusing more on disease prevention and better treatment options over upsell. If they are willing to change, they can become part of the healthcare ecosystem.

Alternatively, the big pharmaceutical companies can be eliminated from the ecosystem. A physician can belong to a provider facility which will receive a medicine supply from a third party manufacturer. This would be a very simple supply chain with minimum hand-offs. Patients will get their medicines faster and at a much lower cost. The mark-up cost of medicine in a complex supply chain in the US can be as high as 3000%. Yes, really—this is not a typo! The cost of medicine can come down significantly by reducing the number of stakeholders in the supply chain network and big pharma can be axed.

The big pharma contributes significantly to the new product introduction to the market through innovative R&D. However, there is a big shift in the way pharmaceutical R&D operates today. The blockbuster drugs (generating at least USD 1 billion revenue annually) are long gone. The cost of drug development is now close to USD 2 billion and only a handful of drugs can return the invested amount. More and more orphan drugs (drugs treating less than 200,000 patients) are being approved and thousands are in the pipeline. On average, about 140 orphan drugs are now under development, which is almost three times the number a decade ago. This indicates that both the pharmaceutical industry and the health authorities have acknowledged the value of medicines for smaller markets and the need to make them more affordable as well as realize a better return on investment.

The age of specialization is back—developing, manufacturing and distributing products to serve a specific patient segment. Companies are focusing on driving personalized medicine to differentiate it from others.

The specialized products do not need an army of sales professionals to sell. The huge debate between spending more money on the sales and marketing as opposed to R&D has to end. The specialty product business can make that possible. It can also help a pharmaceutical company to extend its services to a patient beyond the selling of pills. There are many opportunities to do that—patient education on disease conditions and treatment options, instruction on side effects, reminders to take medicine on time, monitoring and alerting of severe situations and much more. The human intervention aspect along with the medicine will improve patient health significantly over medicine-only treatment. Big pharmaceutical companies need to make this leap as soon as possible.

The cost of healthcare is overly inflated and the cost of medicine alone contributes significantly to this. In 2011, US prescription drug spend was USD 320 billion and patients with insurance spent USD 49 billion on out-of-pocket expenses [2]. The constant increase in spend with the declining economic situation cannot continue—patients cannot afford to spend more and more every year. Things need to change. So what changes will the pharmaceutical industry make?

Patients are spending less on branded drugs and in 2012 the brand medicines spend is decreased by 5% over the previous year [3]. In 2011 the generic market grew by USD 5.6 billion in the US. The major reasons for this are the economic downturn and the availability of quality generic products on the market. The patients have made their choice on using good quality generics over high cost branded drugs.

In summary, the pharmaceutical industry needs to make a decision. It needs to redesign itself to carry on as a viable business in the healthcare ecosystem. The advancement of technology has enabled better treatment options, increased customer demand, changes in drug development and selling pattern, inflation of the cost of healthcare and an increase in out-of-pocket costs for the patient. All these changes will force the pharmaceutical industry to redesign itself.

There has been an imbalance in the growth of the pharmaceutical industry. Growth equals innovation plus productivity—in this equation, growth is flat for the industry and innovation is negative. The growth equation can be made to balance if the industry works towards improving productivity immediately. In the long run they can continue building on innovation-driven growth, but today's solution has to be productivity-driven to make an immediate impact. This is another way the industry can survive through redesign.

The prognosis indicates that large companies with high overheads, process barriers, difficulties with bringing in changes faster and high expectations of profitability can improve in a smaller company set-up. Smaller companies can run smarter and execute nimbler operations. They can have greater flexibility in business strategy, look for targeted business opportunities with focused investment plans, drive specialized product business, and compete within a specific therapy segment as opposed to managing too many broader brands managed by big pharma. They can bring in dedicated services for their customer segments faster. The industry has already made some movement towards this: the split of Abbott branded drug business into AbbVie, and Pfizer's animal health business spin-off Zoetis are sizable examples. The split of Kraft food and Mondelez is another prominent example in the food industry. Very recently, the Covidien spin-off of its pharmaceuticals business, Mallinckrodt, has been added to this list and many more are in talks. The Zoetis spin-off may become a trendsetter in the industry after its huge initial success in exciting the stock market. Eli Lilly, Merck and Sanofi have similar patent cliff challenges to those that Pfizer had and an animal health business such as Pfizer's could be the savior, proving again that "smaller is beautiful".

How will smaller companies be able to solve their current business issues? The key driver of M&A has always been to create a very diversified business. If we go back to the pharmaceutical industry's largest M&A deal, Pfizer & Wyeth, the whole idea was to make Pfizer the most diversified company in the pharmaceutical world. The intention was to meet everyone's need through a single company, but today, the needs are very specialized and can be met better by a specialized service provider. The Figure 1.1 describes the shift from today's big pharma model to smaller companies in the future.

Several smaller companies have shown operational flexibility and smarter innovation and have maintained higher growth. Forrest Labs and Novo Nordisk are good examples in the pharmaceutical industry.

A large pharmaceutical company needs to take several key actions to save its business:

1. Make the business nimble through spin-offs or effect logical separation of specialized business areas. This will simplify overall product supply and make drug delivery easier and less expensive. Specialized product manufacturing can bring in smarter technologies faster to make operations more productive and cost-effective. Use of robots in manufacturing, effective usage of a manufacturing execution system and making the shop-floor operations team more powerful through manufacturing knowledge management systems are all possible for specialized product manufacturing units.

TODAY: Big Pharma	TOMORROW: Smaller Pharma
R&D is unable to produce blockbuster drugs. The development cost has gone over $1B with very little success in return on investment	Drives move away from blockbuster drugs. Orphan drug/ personalized medicine/specialty drugs are the focus. Faster development, low marketing cost, higher RoI
Technology driven innovation is harder to adopt	Focused change management & training to a smaller set of stakeholders to adopt the technology driven innovation such as using robots in manufacturing
Unable to deliver demands of more educated customers including patient, physician, payers & providers	Smaller company will be created to focus on a specific therapy area. Customers will be segmented into a smaller set which will be manageable better
Larger revenue expectation from a brand with the army of sales personnel in the field	Specialty product selling needs only a smaller sales team. They get better access to physicians for detailing. Low cost, high impact sales team.
Unable to improve productivity for higher overhead, complex processes and fear of changes	Smaller companies will be nimble, simplify supply chain for faster delivery to drive productivity improvement across the value chain

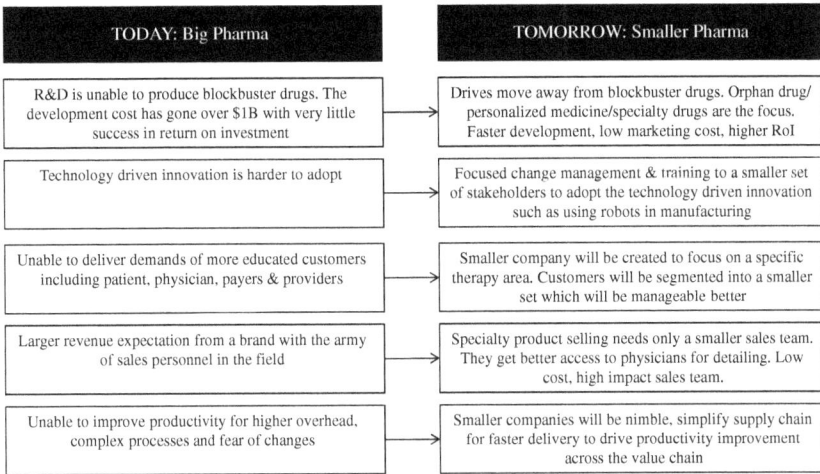

FIGURE 1.1   Shift of big Pharma model.

2. Be more patient centric. Going beyond selling products to take care of patients will make big pharma a part of the healthcare ecosystem. The current binary communication between physician and pharmaceutical company, or physician and patient can only be of limited value; these communications are not optimized. There is a need to create a system of continual tri-party communications. Pharmaceutical companies can create a platform for a specific disease condition or for a product brand through which all stakeholders can share their views and benefit from each other's knowledge. The pharmaceutical industry's closed loop marketing strategy using integrated and interactive multi-channel marketing can increase interaction with the customers, going beyond physicians. A small and nimble company can make this happen faster and better than a gigantic global pharmaceutical company.

3. Make R&D more predictable and increase return on investment. This can be achieved by concentrating on specialty drugs, personalized medicine and orphan drugs. The investment will be lower per molecule, will make compounds more predictable and help generate more revenue. R&D cannot remain within the company's four walls. The crowd-sourcing of ideas, methods, parts of the target compounds, safety insights, drug knowledge and data can eliminate several years of unproductive work for a company. The company needs to interact more with the world outside it, to let the world in, to make it a better, more effective company. This has been

proven in several pharmaceutical companies and other industries as well. The P&G Connect + Develop, Audi Production Award, SAP Co-Innovation Lab, HP, Nokia, Cisco—many of these companies have set examples for the pharmaceutical industry [4]. The good news is that Pfizer, GSK, Medtronic, Novartis and others have embarked on open innovation initiatives— this may not be on a bigger scale but they are moving forward.

4. Employ specialized sales teams to sell your specialized product. A large, multi-product company sales team has to deal with too much conflicting information as it moves from brand to brand or from place to place. The use of digital and mobile technologies can make them even more efficient.

5. Allow part of your business to be run by third parties to free up capital investment. A small company can retain the product-specific knowledge-based work within the company and offload support functions to third parties. If we break the work into "find", "produce", "supply", "sell", "comply" and "manage", there are several parts that can be executed by specialized third parties. A specialized executer will ensure that its segment is run at the highest level of maturity. This will help it to operate without much capital locked into support areas to increase free cash flow. This not only helps to operate a nimbler company, but increases brand equity to the shareholders, making the company a lot more attractive for investment. As companies focus more on emerging markets, external collaboration with local companies in emerging markets makes it much easier to establish "going global with local connections".

6. In emerging markets, and in smaller and underdeveloped countries, regulations will increasingly become more complex for local as well as globally run operations. A smaller company may be able to operate in a much smarter way to meet all the regulations and run the company more effectively in the world's compliance maze.

These smaller and more nimble companies will need to be connected virtually to avoid information silos. Using information technology has become the driving force behind this new operating model. Several other industries have made this choice already and the pharmaceutical industry will also benefit from the use of technology to make the redesign work as long as it becomes a prime design principle. These changes may not make the pharmaceutical industry indispensable, but they will solidify its existence by delivering a much better service to their shareholders than they do today.

The innovation and financial power of the pharmaceutical industry is currently not very high. It is under severe pressure for many reasons—some are internal to the company and many are external. It can redesign operations to overcome internal challenges which are under their control, but the external causes need bigger changes to be made to the way the businesses are run.

The damage to the big pharmaceutical companies is not yet beyond repair. Together, business and technology will be able to bring in changes better, faster and to a level acceptable to all. It does, however, need much more cooperation between the two sides. This can come about through a better understanding of the other side's functions. The value chain of a pharmaceutical business needs to be understood by the technologists; similarly, business executives should have basic IT knowledge to appreciate and help each other reach their individual and combined goals.

Chapters 2 and 3 in this book give basic information about the pharmaceutical business side for technologists, followed by the basics of technology for business executives. Once a successful business and IT foundation has been created, we discuss seven themes in Chapter 4 which will transform the pharmaceutical business. These themes are in line with the recommendations made earlier in this chapter. Chapter 5 concludes with the design of value structure of an organization and how to measure values.

Chapter 2

The Pharmaceutical Value Chain—An Introduction

The definition of a drug by the Food & Drug Administration (FDA) is: a substance recognized by an official pharmacopoeia or formulary; a substance intended for use in the diagnosis, cure, mitigation, treatment, or prevention of disease; a substance (other than food) intended to affect the structure or any function of the body; or a substance intended for use as a component of a medicine but not a device or a component, part or accessory of a device [5].

A global, research-based pharmaceutical organization manufactures and sells branded products and over the counter products. There are contract manufacturing organizations (CMO) that are responsible for manufacturing products for other pharmaceutical companies and there are companies who manufacture generic products—products that are out of patent, as a lower cost alternative to the branded products. While these companies have different business models and need to refine various functional areas to meet their needs, this chapter will focus on the big pharmaceutical business.

The pharmaceutical value chain has five broader segments— Research & Development, Manufacturing and Supply Chain, Sales and Marketing, Regulatory and Corporate Functions. These areas are further divided into functional areas represented in Figure 2.1. Most research-based pharmaceutical organizations are broadly divided into these segments.

Drug discovery and development follows a long and uneven path, and every drug follows its own road. During the long process of drug development, the use of the drug may change and another use is discovered, either intentionally or by accident. Retrovir (AZT) was first studied as an anticancer drug in the 1960s with disappointing results

Pharma's Prescription. http://dx.doi.org/10.1016/B978-0-12-407662-4.00002-7

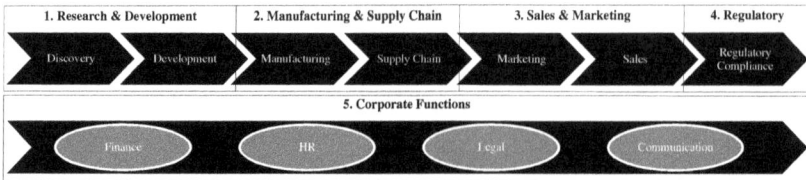

FIGURE 2.1   Pharmaceutical value-chain.

[6a]. Twenty years later, researchers discovered that the drug could treat AIDS, and the US FDA approved the drug, manufactured by GlaxoSmithKline, for that purpose in 1987. The HN2 is still classified as a schedule 1 weapon by the Chemical Weapons Convention—can you imagine it is one of the best-known nitrogen mustards, the first anticancer chemotherapy drug? Now, the well-known and exciting one—Viagra (Sildenafil citrate)—started life as a plain old UK92480, a new treatment for angina, a heart condition that constricts the vessels that supply the heart with blood [6b]. Sildenafil citrate didn't perform well in trials, but the molecule did give patients a side effect—penile erection. That's how the first ever oral treatment for erectile dysfunction was introduced in 1998.

The pharmaceutical industry doesn't get lucky all the time though—not all side effects are beneficial. There are many incidents of drugs that are recalled from the market by the health authorities because of adverse side effects. While many drugs are developed by accident, the R&D researchers don't rely on accidents to determine the fate of their research. They follow a very structured approach to discover and develop drugs and design them carefully to treat a disease condition or improve well-being. Most drug candidates in the animal trial never go for the human trial and health authority's review. Only a few drug candidates go through the agency's rigorous evaluation process including the design of clinical trials, test methods, test results, side effects and the manufacturing methods.

The 14 Steps in Drug Discovery and Development

There are 14 high-level steps for a pharmaceutical company to develop a drug, get it approved by the health authorities (e.g. FDA) and make it available to the end users (see Figure 2.2).

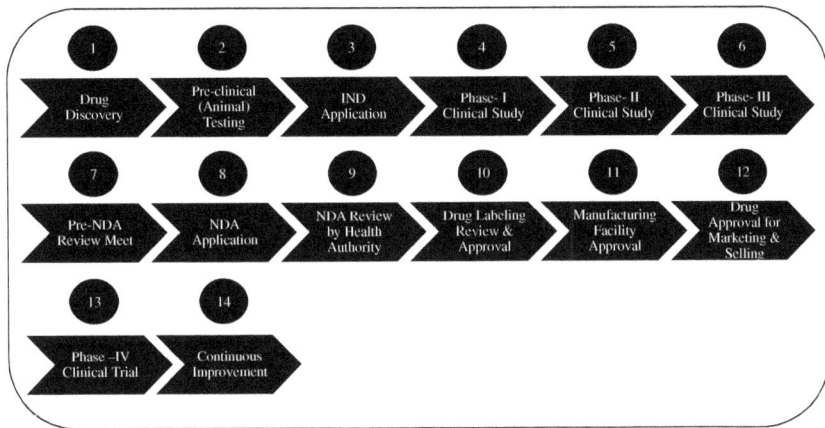

FIGURE 2.2   Pharmaceutical R&D steps.

DRUG DISCOVERY

Drug discovery is the process of discovering chemical or biological molecules with medicinal values or molecules that have an influence on how an organ works. These molecules are purposed to treat a specific disease condition or improve well-being. This critical function has undergone phenomenal torsions over the years—right from the heavy-duty, laboratory-based drug discovery to the predictive, in-silico-based drug discovery model. This shift has made the process more productive, simpler, shorter and predictable. Information Technology (IT) plays a significant role in making this turn effectively.

Drug discovery is a continuous, evolving process with many dynamic attributes. However, we are starting with a conventional drug discovery process that is easy to understand for beginners—business stakeholders outside R&D functions and IT practitioners who want to interact with R&D scientists to execute technology projects. The diagram in Figure 2.3 represents the drug discovery process.

The drug discovery process starts with the understanding of disease states and tries to identify functional changes that cause a disease (genes, proteins, tissues, environmental conditions, etc.). This step is to find out how the disease occurs and how molecular level instabilities produce certain symptoms that are visible to individuals as a disease symptom. When drug discovery scientists understand this mechanism, they then find a protein that controls this condition. This protein is called the target and the whole process is known as **Target Identification**.

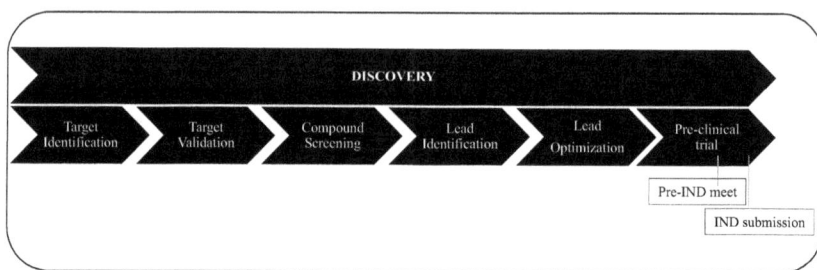

FIGURE 2.3   Drug discovery steps.

Once a target is identified, making the decision to develop a drug against the particular target is a huge commitment of time and money from a pharmaceutical company. The development takes over 10 years and it can cost over USD 1 billion. Most drug candidates fail at a later stage of the drug development process due to various safety and efficacy reasons caused by poor selection of a target. So scientists take a very careful approach to validate this target through several techniques. This is the stage to find out the role of a target and the effects of manipulating a target candidate (e.g. What if I knock a gene out?). This stage is called **Target Validation**.

Researchers look for several aspects of the target to find a drug compound—what part of the protein really acts (the active site); what compound can bind to this active site which can make the protein dysfunctional; can we actually create the compound which binds to the target, etc. They look for ways to prevent the proper functioning of the target. If the target (protein) can't function properly the disease condition doesn't appear. The scientists sift through the huge volume of existing data in search of thousands of chemical or biochemical compounds that can potentially block the function of this protein. Pharmaceutical companies have libraries of chemical or biochemical compounds, and several of these compounds are hypothetically structured using software applications based on the protein binding properties. The process of finding the compound which can potentially inhibit the target is called **Compound Screening**.

There are certain tests conducted to assess the performance of a screened compound. The testing process is known as **Assay**. This is a test to determine how a compound inhibits or stimulates a biochemical or biological mechanism on a given target. Assays could be of cell-based/in vitro assays where the drug demonstrates cell proliferation or cell death, cell metabolism or intracellular signaling, receptor binding or gene reporter assays. It can also be of in vivo/animal models assays where this involves animal models or transgenic animals for testing.

Using robotics, the High-Throughput Screening (HTS) allows conducting millions of pharmacological tests very quickly. The potential candidates are re-tested for assay and result reproducibility through different assay types. In general, of the thousands of compounds tested, barely 1% will pass this test to move into the next stage. Information Technology plays a large role in today's compound assay techniques to make the process more productive.

The next step is to find out Structure Activity Relationship (SAR). Additional tests are performed to determine selectivity, potency and mechanism of action of the compounds. The compounds that are specific and selective on a therapeutic target, absorb well and with minimum side effects, are taken into the next level of the drug discovery process as lead candidates and the process is termed as **Lead Identification**.

The leads are further characterized and validated for effectiveness and toxicity before they are tested on animals. Only 10–20% of the lead compound survives through this further scrutiny which is known as **Lead Optimization**. Lead optimization ensures effectiveness, low toxicity and higher absorption compounds. Several technologies used in lead identification can be used in lead optimization as well. Microarrays have been used in genomics/proteomics approaches for gene expression profiling and target validation. Bioinformatics is used for target identification and validation. Antisense technologies enable sequence-based gene knockdown at the RNA level. The drug candidates successfully completing the lead optimization stage move into the pre-clinical (animal) trial process.

When Lorie was born in 2009, she was born with SMA—Spinal Muscular Atrophy—a genetic disorder that makes muscles progressively weaken, paralyses and creates respiratory failure. Her family was devastated. They were told she wouldn't be able to move her muscles—wouldn't sit up, crawl or walk. She wouldn't have the ability to swallow and breathe on her own. One out of every 6,000 births may lack a key biological ingredient, a critical protein essential for the survival of its neurons, which sends nerve signals from the spinal cord to muscles. This is the reason for SMA, the leading genetic cause of death of children under the age of two in the United States. It's a methodical killer—with no cure or serious hope for a treatment until a laboratory at Columbia University could identify the gene responsible for this deficiency. They have used high-throughput screening (HTS) and a new software program to make the impossible possible. This is an extraordinary example of improving pharmaceutical research using technology. Spinal Muscular Atrophy: http://cumc.columbia.edu/research/animal/Muscular_Atrophy.html.

Pre-Clinical (Animal) Trials

About 20–30 lead candidates are selected to move into a pre-clinical trial. The pre-clinical trial is to find the answer to the question: "Is this compound safe to proceed to human trials"?

This stage of research begins to test the product safety in animals before clinical trials—testing on humans—can begin. The fundamental aspect in safety assessment is called PK/PD (Pharmacokinetics/ Pharmacodynamics). The PK study tells us what the body does to the drug substance and PD tells us what the drug substance does to the human body. Animal testing helps measure how much of the drug is absorbed into the blood, how it is broken down chemically, its toxicity level, its metabolites, and how quickly the drug components are excreted out of the human body. This is called the ADME study where the Absorption, Distribution, Metabolism and Excretion of the drug are measured. The entire study needs to follow very specific regulatory guidelines established by the health authorities, e.g. Food & Drug Administration (FDA) in the US, European Medical Agency (EMA) in the EU or Therapeutic Drug Administration (TGA) in Australia, to name a few. The health authorities try to understand several aspects of the drug under investigation including pharmacological profile and acute toxicity. The clinical trial duration determines what short-term toxicity duration has to be established, ranging between two weeks to three months. The bioavailability study of the drug is an essential parameter to be considered for calculating the dosage for non-intravenous administration and the optimum dose range via dose response curve. The entire pre-clinical study of a new drug takes about two to three years. The experiments are performed in both in-vitro and in-vivo conditions. The in-vitro tests are conducted using components of an organism that have been isolated from their usual biological surroundings and in-vivo experimentation uses a whole, living organism.

Animal testing in the pharmaceutical industry has been reduced lately for ethical reasons. However, we still don't have an alternate option to animals for the similar anatomy and physiology required in development. This may soon change if the virtual animal or human organ creation using various technologies becomes reality. The fast development and maturity of the 3D printing of human organs may make this possible soon.

These days, prior to clinical studies, pharmaceutical companies may meet with health authorities to make decisions on pre-clinical studies based on bioactivity and product safety for administration. This meeting, referred to as the **Pre-IND meeting**, is useful at this early development stage for discussion on the trial of any special requests, e.g. orphan drug approval before

IND (Investigational New Drug) submission. The IND is the documented evidence of pre-clinical trials and the formal process to inform trial results to the health authority before moving into the clinical trial stage.

The **IND submission** typically outlines the following:

- The pharmacological and toxicology results
- Chemistry and manufacturing information
- Detailed protocol of the proposed clinical studies—to ensure that subjects are not exposed to unnecessary risks
- The details of the Sponsor/CRO who would be responsible to conduct the study; this also includes the investigator's qualification and eligibility to conduct the trial.

Once the IND is submitted to the regulatory body (e.g. FDA), it becomes effective in 30 days if not disapproved before that. More details on IND submission are described in the Regulatory Compliance section (see page 53).

Technology Tie-Up

While the discovery process looks simple, the industry didn't do well and there are significant opportunities to improve. The good news is that the industry has more research knowledge and data than ever before. Several predictive analytics tools are available and can use this data to make discovery more productive. However, this analysis process is struggling because over 80% of company data is unstructured and up to 50% of information isn't indexed and is not easy to find later.

When Jenny, a bench scientist in Groton, Connecticut, USA wants to find toxicity information of a compound using standard databases she can't get the optimum output—not all the information comes up to her analysis as it is not indexed. This is a huge loss of information that the pharmaceutical industry will soon be able to avoid with the help of data and information management technologies and an analytics foundation using big data solutions.

When we worked with one of the top five food and beverage manufacturing companies who were trying to improve the food value in their product through genetically modified raw material, it was quickly decided to use an open innovation technique to source more ideas and existing research information from the outside world. While finding the external partners wasn't so challenging, it was more difficult to find the right information, standardize data, share data and information securely between companies. This became an even bigger challenge when we found various levels of information management maturity within this diverse set of partners. But the information technology came as a big help. It not only helped to standardize the data creation and transmission, and analyzing of data for reproducibility at different laboratories, but also helped speed up the process by sourcing the right information right away to eliminate any need for re-work. The research team's productivity was improved up to 40%, data availability was increased by 100% and previous experiment data was made available online for easy access by their lab scientists globally. This was done in little over a year and wouldn't have been possible so fast without the help of information technology.

The use of big data technology helps in managing and effectively using data for more accurate research prediction. This helps us to identify the right candidate more quickly. We are experiencing a foundational shift in medical discovery in which "we react to a disease after it's happened" to the "we act to prevent illness". The medicines will be highly personalized through the frenzied rate of discovery related to genomics. There will be a need to define, create, manage and analyze personal data along with the huge load of research data in order to create the magical solution. The big data analytics will play a central role in this shift. This will free up over USD 100 billion from the R&D spend in the pharmaceutical industry by managing the industry's data explosion better. A fully integrated R&D (internally and externally), real-time visibility of clinical trials and monitoring marketed drugs for adverse events more effectively will make this possible. Molplex and Microsoft Research Connections have proved this in a pre-clinical study. They have used over 10,000 chemical structures to create over 750,000 predictive structure activity relationships. They have used their computational platform to validate this data set to narrow the number to about 23,000 models that scientists can look at further [7]. This eliminates over 97% of the bandwidth and possibly the cost too.

Another area of improvement is to reduce the "fear of failure". Technology-driven iterative and predictive computer-based studies eliminate the chance of failure in a later stage. The computer-based algorithm can work wonders if used with limited scale lab data to predict the success in a later stage. With increased knowledge on the human gene, disease pathways and other drug mechanism of action, it's possible to mimic virtual humans to analyze compounds for higher predictability in compound screening.

The IND submission process takes a long time which can be shorted by 50% through effective use of technologies. There are several authoring tools, online review systems and electronic submission techniques that in combination can create the impact needed. More details on this are given in Chapter 4: Scream With Mouth Shut—Global Compliance Strategy.

DEVELOPMENT

Not all drug candidates survive through the pre-clinical phase—only three to four drug candidates from the pre-clinical phase become successful and move into a clinical trial. A clinical study involves human volunteers (also called subjects) and needs great precautions taken. When a new drug is developed, the investigators try to establish the safety and efficacy of the drug candidate by measuring outcomes in the clinical trial participants. For example, investigators may give a drug to participants with high blood pressure to see if their blood pressure decreases. It starts with a small and healthy population, before trying a larger population base.

The entire trial is broken down into multiple phases based on purpose, subject condition, duration, etc. The chart in Figure 2.4 describes the various clinical trial phases.

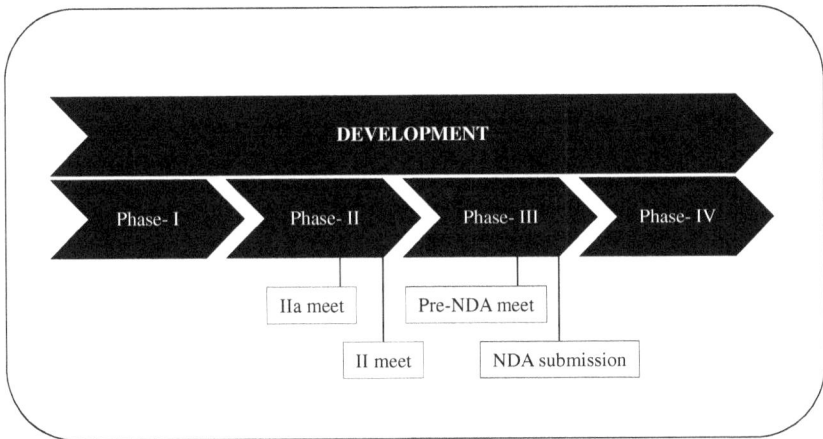

FIGURE 2.4   Drug development phases.

Phase I: Studies that are usually conducted with healthy volunteers (subjects) and to emphasize safety. The goal is to find out what the drug's most frequent and serious side effects are and how the drug is metabolized and excreted [8].

Phase II: This phase proves the effectiveness (whether the drug works in people who have a certain disease or condition). For example, participants receiving the drug may be compared with similar participants receiving a different treatment, usually an inactive substance (placebo) or another drug. Safety continues to be evaluated, and short-term adverse events are studied.

Phase III: This study phase gathers more information about safety and effectiveness by studying different populations and different dosages and by using the drug in combination with other drugs.

Phase IV: This occurs after the health authority of the country where the product launch is taking place has approved the drug for marketing. This phase gathers additional information about a drug's safety, efficacy, or optimal use while it is used by the patients

The chart in Table 2.1 describes various phases and their key study parameters.

TABLE 2.1

Phases	Study Purpose	# Subjects (Human Volunteers)	Trial Length
Phase I: Drug is tested on healthy volunteers to determine toxicity relative to dose and to screen for unexpected side effects	First use in humans to find safe dose Safety, Metabolism and Excretion of the drug (ADME), bioactivity, Drug–drug interaction	Tens of healthy volunteers or very ill patients	6 to 12 months
Phase II: Drug is tested on a small group of patients to see if it has any beneficial effect and to determine the dose level needed for this effect	Short-term side effects and efficacy	Hundreds of subjects with indication	12 to 24 months
Phase III: Drug is tested on a much larger group of patients and compared with existing treatments and with a placebo	Safety and efficacy Basis for labeling, new formulations	Thousands of subjects with indication	12 to 36 months
Phase IV: Marketed drugs are monitored for the side effects	New indications, QoL, surveillance	Drug is exposed to thousands of diverse population groups across the globe	12 to 60 months

How Clinical Trials are Executed

As the clinical trial involves human volunteers, it is highly regulated. This needs to follow approved processes and standards as defined by health authorities, executed by trained professionals, reviewed and approved by independent bodies and, more importantly, needs to ensure the welfare of human volunteers in the trial.

The human volunteers are protected by laws and best practices throughout the entire clinical trial process. This includes "THE NUREMBERG CODE—Permissible Medical Experiments" which warrants the physician to experiment with specific purposes and protects human volunteers. The genesis of the Nuremberg Code was the Nuremberg Doctors' Trial of 1946 when an American military tribunal opened criminal proceedings against 23 leading German physicians and administrators for their willing participation in war crimes and crimes against humanity [9]. In Nazi Germany, these physicians planned and enacted the "Euthanasia" Program, the systematic killing of those they deemed "unworthy of life". The victims included the mentally retarded, the institutionalized mentally ill, and the physically impaired. In addition, during World War II, these physicians conducted pseudoscientific medical experiments utilizing thousands of concentration camp prisoners without their consent. Most died or were permanently crippled as a result. After almost 140 days of proceedings, including the testimony of 85 witnesses and the submission of almost 1,500 documents, the American judges pronounced their verdict on August 20, 1947. Sixteen of the doctors were found guilty. Seven were sentenced to death. This trial also helped to define permissible medical experiments by medical professionals.

The broad outline of the clinical trial process has the following steps:

1. Protocol Design
2. Study Initiation including Patient Recruitment & Enrolment
3. Study Execution
4. Study Report
5. Study Closure

Two major activities that go across the clinical trial process are: (1) Quality Management and (2) Project Management & Governance. Typically, a clinical trial requires the active involvement of various stakeholders, in various combinations, including Sponsor (mostly pharmaceutical companies), Investigator (Physician), Clinical Research Associate (CRA), Clinical Data Manager (CDM), Clinical Data Programmer (CDP),

Statistician, Clinical Research Organization (CRO), Independent Review Board (IRB), and regulatory authorities (e.g. FDA).

The chart in Figure 2.5 provides an overview of all the process and stakeholder contributions.

The **Sponsor** (drug manufacturer) takes responsibility for the drug trials and approval. The first responsibility is to initiate a trial after going through health authority approval and also **IRB** (Institutional Review Board) approval. The Sponsor manages the entire clinical trial process, either using their internal resources or outsourcing to companies who are specialized in clinical trial activities such as trial execution, data management, reporting and submissions. The **Contract Research Organization** (CRO) is one such company who helps sponsor companies to execute clinical trials. The **Investigator** team (Physician, Nurse, Pharmacist, and Laboratory Technician) conducts the clinical trial. The investigator should be a qualified person, well trained and experienced, to execute clinical trials. The responsibilities of the investigator include obtaining approval of IRB, eligible trial subjects recruitment, obtaining an informed consent form from trial participants, trial planning and management, trial execution, communication with the sponsor and the IRB. The IRB ensures that the people involved in the process will be safe and

Stakeholder \ Function	Protocol Design	Study Initiation	Study Execution	Study Report	Study Closure
	Quality Management				
	Project Management & Governance				
Sponsor/CRA	• Protocol design & approval • Define SOPs • Identify CROs	• Compensation for subjects & Investigators • Conduct study qualification visit	• Periodic visits during trial/audits • Adverse report handling • Trial termination	• Submit the final reports for regulatory evaluation (NDA)	• Prepare for audit by FDA/respond to queries prior to approval of the NDA.
CRO	• NA	• Patient recruitment • Recruit Investigators • Identify trial sites • Set up CDMS/CTMS	• Acquire data • Manage Central Labs • Monitor study sites	• Study monitoring & reporting • AE/SAE reconciliation	• Assist in Audit • Archiving of documents
Investigator	• NA	• Ensure availability of adequate & trained study staff • Store & handle study drug/information • Obtain written and dated protocol, informed consent form and more	• Provide ongoing medical care • Documentation of trial procedures (Study file, source documents, CRFs) • Inform patient/ IRB in case of premature termination	• Provide summary of study results to IRB • Report AEs/SAEs	• Archiving of documents • Notify IRB on study completion & submit a final report
Subject	• NA	• Informed consent form signature	• Ensure to visit the Trail site at pre-defined interval, • Religiously follow the protocol defined with respect to consuming study drug • Report any side effect to the Investigator		
Data Manager	• NA	• Write CRF/ eCRF • Design database, validation, Thesaurus, etc	• Data entry/Verification • Generate queries & update resolution	• AE/SAE Reconciliation • Database Audit • Draft Study report (Medical writing)	• Database Lock/closure • Bookmarking and Hyper linking of the final report
IT & Statistician	• NA	• Set up Programming environment • Map source data to standards • Statistical analysis plan (Interim and final) • Sample size calculation	• Programming for all Safety and efficacy tables • Create analysis datasets	• Review of reports, tables by clinical and biometric teams • Issue of final biometrics tables and report text	• Database Freeze • Submission ready files
IRB/ Independent Ethic committee	• Review proposed protocol • Validate Investigator qualification • Review recruitment documents (e.g. advertisement)	• Review Informed consent forms and subject payment	• Conduct continuing review of each ongoing study at least once a year • Safe guarding the rights, safety and well being of all study subjects		

FIGURE 2.5　Clinical trial stakeholder contribution.

their protection rights of participating on consent, withdrawing from the trial and getting information about each step of the trial are protected. The **Clinical Data Management, Programmer and Statistician** teams ensure the right data quality and analyzing of data as per the protocol. **Health Authorities** of all countries where the sponsor wishes to market the product review the study report before approving the drug marketability. Studies can be done in professional settings, academic or private settings. The clinical trial information for a drug is made public in the US.

A growing emphasis has been made on the standardization of the workflow to ensure the reproducibility and reliability of the global trial.

Protocol Design Standardization

The clinical trial design is very important to establish data integrity and credibility of the information in a study. The study should focus on finding a treatment option or improving the well-being of a large population through various study parameters including product safety, benefits and risks. The exception is with the Orphan Drug approval in which case the drug can be specific to a smaller number of the population (less than 200,000) and pharmaceutical companies get the right to market the drug exclusively for seven years. Protocols must be pre-approved for the endpoint—what would the trial prove? Health authorities or the scientific community do not accept post-trial claims that were not mentioned in the protocol—"cherry-picking" is not allowed.

The Tuskegee syphilis experiment was an infamous clinical study conducted between 1932 and 1972 by the US Public Health Service to study the natural progression of untreated syphilis in rural black men who thought they were receiving free healthcare from the US government [10]. Investigators enrolled a total of 600 impoverished sharecroppers from Macon County, Alabama in the study: 399 had previously contracted syphilis before the study began, and 201 without the disease. For participating in the study, the men were given free medical care, meals and free burial insurance. They were never told they had syphilis, nor were they ever treated for it. According to the Center for Disease Control, the men were told they were being treated for "bad blood", a local term for various illnesses that include syphilis, anemia and fatigue. The 40-year study was controversial for reasons related to ethical standards, primarily because researchers knowingly failed to treat patients appropriately even after knowing the treatment options. Since 1981, the Health Authorities appointed the IRB to review and approve study protocol before inception of the trial.

A study protocol may consist of the following:

1. Study contact details (Sponsor, Principal Investigator, IRB Leader, Project Leader)
2. Study objective, background and rationale
3. Plan and procedures (study type, clinic visit schedule, assessment plan by visit, study population, subject inclusion and exclusion criteria with justification, criteria for study discontinuation, investigational products and treatment details, treatment schedule, randomization, storage and accountability, allowed medication and compliance)
4. Study measurements and end goals (primary and secondary safety endpoints, measurements at each visit, adverse events, ECG/EKG, laboratory investigations, haematology, clinical chemistry, blood levels of active constituents, measurements recorded daily in diary)
5. Statistical methods (determination of sample size, statistical analysis protocol, reporting, changes to the protocol)
6. Ethics (ethics review, ethical conduct of the study, subject information and consent, subject data protection, insurance and indemnity)
7. Data management, data quality assurance, programming, reporting
8. Timeline and termination
9. References.

Study Initiation

This stage includes identification/section of investigators, trial sites, set up of Clinical Data Management System (CDMS) and Clinical Trial Management System (CTMS), CRF standardization, patient recruitment and enrollment, collection of signed and dated informed consent forms.

CRF Standardization

A Clinical Report Form (CRF) is a regulated document to collect data from the subjects and must include design, usability, data entry, data quality, validity, accuracy and privacy. This data can be collected on paper or electronically. The study design protocol governs which data should be collected in the CRF and specific analysis milestones during the trial execution and at the study closure.

Patient Selection/Recruitment Standardization

After the investigator is selected and trained on the protocol, the patient selection/recruitment begins based on the inclusion and exclusion criteria as defined in the protocol. The protocol helps define the target population, and demographic data is used to define the subject recruitment target. The patient recruitment strategies are sent to the IRB or ethics committee for approval. Once the plans are approved, the subjects are recruited as per the approved plan. Methods may include web, print advertisement, radio announcements, using patient database, television marketing, physician referral and direct mail. Once subjects are identified, their data is collected and screened for their eligibility before enrolling in the study. The eligibility criteria may include age, gender, ethnic background, state of health, and absence or presence of specific diseases that are related to the clinical trial. There are several technology tools to help the recruitment process by mixing and matching patient data with that of existing databases. The subject enrollment communication needs to be sent with the detailed information on the study, including potential risks, or the potential subject can approach the physician or their delegated study staff to understand this better. After the enrollment process, the subject needs to complete the informed consent process. This process details the study protocol and the risks and benefits. Each enrolled subject must sign an Informed Consent Form (ICF). Enrolled subjects are then randomly grouped and specific activity plans and schedules are created for the subjects and the investigators.

The Informed Consent Form should include explanations of the following:

- The trial involves research
- Purpose of the trial
- Trial procedures including any invasive procedures
- Subject responsibility
- Risks and benefits
- Expected benefits
- Alternative procedure or courses available for treatment
- Compensation and treatment availability during any trial injury
- Person to contact during emergency
- Approximate number of subjects involved in the trial
- Expected duration of subject's participation.

Study Execution

This stage is based on the subjects' visit schedule and tracks their condition after drug administration. Study data is collected accurately and stored in the database. Several technology systems are used to enter, analyze and monitor subject data. Lab tests are done to monitor the effects of the study drug on the subjects. The study starts with First Patient First Visit (FPFV) up to Last Patient Last Visit (LPLV). There are parallel processes including trial monitoring and follow-up visits. The subjects are enrolled either as in-patient or will be required to visit the investigator as specified in the protocol. There are several important roles to execute the report and manage the trial process. The Clinical Research Coordinator (CRC) is responsible for subject scheduling, subject visit management, compliance checks, CRF completion and reporting to various stakeholders. The clinical data manager is responsible for data entry, data cleansing, data validation, etc. The investigator examines the subject during scheduled visits and records the symptoms or conditions. The investigator prescribes medication, draws samples and orders tests. The pharmacist dispatches the drugs prescribed by the investigator. Lab analysts test the clinical trial samples and record results in the system. While the data gets recorded and is analyzed at certain intervals, any serious adverse events must be reported as soon as they occur.

One of the worst side effects in medical history is that of Thalidomide [11]. Thalidomide first entered the German market in 1957 as an over the counter remedy and was marketed in over 40 countries in the next couple of years. Thalidomide was entered on the market as a tranquilizer and sleeping pill but its off-label prescription become very popular too. Doctors all over the world started giving this medicine to pregnant women for morning sickness. But this practice led to a very serious adverse drug reaction to the fetus. In 1961, doctors began to associate this so-called harmless compound with severe birth defects in the babies delivered. Between 1957 and 1962, thousands of children were born with severe malformations including Phocomelia, because their mothers had taken thalidomide during pregnancy. Phocomelia is a birth disorder with very short or absent long bones and flipper-like appearance of hands and sometimes feet.

Study Reporting

A study report needs to be created and sent to the health authorities, sponsors, IRB and principal investigators to report the trial status, data, any special events, etc. Various people involved in different roles in the study create reports at different stages of the trial. The submission documents need to be created and submitted in the country where the drug is intended to be marketed.

Study Closing

The end of a clinical trial is always defined in the protocol. All the trial data must be secured and locked as per the regulations. The data lock is a predetermined date and time after which no new data can be submitted to support NDA submission. After the database has been locked the data cannot be modified. The locked data is then used for statistical analysis and the final trial results are sent to the health authorities. Study closing involves the following:

- Informing the IRB/IEC that all participant follow-up has been completed
- Tracking and documenting progress towards meeting all requirements
- Resolving all outstanding monitoring findings/queries
- Ensuring that all data management queries, drug safety and coding have been addressed.

Quality Control (QC)

The success of a clinical trial depends on the data quality as all the analysis and inferences are drawn from the data recorded in the system. Clinical data quality standards are established by various government and industry forums. The Clinical Data Interchange Standards Consortium (CDISC) is a data standard widely used in the industry [12]. The overall quality assurance and control is done through process definition, roles and responsibilities and independent audits at specific intervals. A clinical trial can be suspended or terminated by the IRB under 21 CFR 56 if the trial is not conducted as per the IRB's requirements or the trial has done some unexpected serious harm to the subjects.

Project Management and Governance

A clinical trial consists of managing several processes, a large number of stakeholders, thousands of diversified subjects, a huge amount of data and a large global technology infrastructure. All the activities need to be performed in compliance with regulatory guidelines. A dedicated and strong project management plan and governance touch points are a fundamental part of a successful clinical trial program.

Pre-NDA Review Meet

This is a meeting between the sponsor and Food & Drug Administration (FDA) to uncover any major issues, identify studies that will show the effectiveness and acquaint the FDA with the product information. The NDA typically outlines:

- A detailed summary of the clinical trials
- A submission format and data presentation method.

This is the document complied by the sponsor and tells the complete story of the drug, starting from its discovery, composition/ingredients, results of the animal studies, PK/PD data, summary of clinical tests, safety report, toxicology results, manufacturing process, packaging and labeling details.

The FDA would have 60 days to complete their preliminary review after receiving the application. If the NDA is insufficiently completed, the FDA issues a Refuse to File Letter explaining the reason behind the rejection. The FDA uses various predefined criteria to determine if a product takes a standard approval process or a priority review. They communicate their decision through the 74-day letter. The standard FDA review takes about 10 months whereas a priority review gets completed in six months.

Drug Labeling Review and Approval

The US Federal Food, Drug and Cosmetic Act (FFDCA) defines "labeling" as all labels and other written, printed or graphic matter upon any article or any of its containers or wrappers, or accompanying such an article. The term "accompanying" is interpreted liberally to mean more than physical association with the food product. It extends to posters, tags, pamphlets, circulars, booklets, brochures, instructions, websites, etc. Around 22% of the detentions in the USA are due to a labeling mistake. The FDA has a stringent guideline on labeling described in 21 CFR Part 201 Subparts A and C. The labeling ideally constitutes the following:

- Name and place of manufacturing, packer or distributer
- National drug code numbers
- Adequate directions for use
- Statement of ingredients
- Prominence on the required label statements
- Location of expiry date
- Control number to be depicted completely
- Warning statements
- Bar code labeling requirements to be met
- Misleading statements to be avoided, etc.

Manufacturing Facility Approval

The FDA ensures that the drug manufacturing plant is compliant with the regulatory requirements in the following ways:

- Domestic and foreign manufacturing plants are inspected regularly by the inspectors to ensure that they are compliant with Current Good Manufacturing Practice (cGMP)

- The regulatory bodies also inspect the drugs from retail stores, warehouse, etc. and evaluate the complaints received from consumers, doctors, nurses, etc. This information helps them to identify the need for enforcement action, scrutiny, educational outreach, new guidance/regulations.

Drug Approved for Marketing and Selling

The regulatory body approves the following types of drugs:

- Prescription or Branded Drugs—This has to follow the stringent process as mentioned above including the discovery, animal studies, IND submission, clinical trials and finally NDA submission for review and approval
- Generic Drugs—These are also referred to as copycat drugs. They are similar to an existing patent drug. The manufacturers have to submit an Abbreviated New Drug Application (ANDA). As an existing drug is already available in the market, the review by the regulatory body would be typically longer
- Over the Counter (OTC) Drugs—The regulatory body has identified a few drugs which are free to market without any supervision/prescription. These are referred to as OTC Drugs and typically marketed as an OTC Drug monograph (this includes the indication for the drug, dosage, etc). Those that comply with the monograph may be marketed without regulatory clearance. However, those that don't fall under the monograph will have to follow the regular NDA submission for review and approval.

R&D Improvement Opportunities and Use of Technologies

The whole process of developing and introducing a new drug costs close to USD 2 billion; and the industry spends nearly 100 billion in a year in R&D. The bad news is that only 20% of marketed drugs can recover the R&D spend. This imposes additional price pressure on the product to do well in the market.

A delay in clinical development can cost over USD 10 million/month, which can make the drug development cost skyrocket. Unfortunately over 72% of clinical trials overrun by several months. The largest spend area is managing data. Subject data collection, analysis, governance, reporting and archival process contributes to about 30% of the overall development cost. However, this area can be improved significantly through effective use of information technology.

Another area of concern is the non-compliance of subject. Over 50% of the subjects do not continue into a clinical trial, which costs USD 10,000-15,000 to recruit a new. This also delays the trial. The non-compliance costs the pharmaceutical industry over USD 30 billion.

Improvement opportunities are plenty. The industry needs an end to end solution to manage the entire development process, data, stakeholders, information and submission to the health authorities. This "drug development in a box" will need to manage the development process holistically. An integrated technology platform which manages the following key components will ensure success:

- Clinical trial management
- Subject recruiting and management
- Investigator recruitment and planning
- Data management
- Clinical supply management
- Lab management
- Study reports
- Submission management
- Predictive analytics

This may sound like development Holy Grail, but the platform-based solution can create an end to end solution by integrating several niche solution components.

While advising a large CRO (Clinical Research Organization) I found the appetite for a consolidated solution by all the stakeholders—internal and external to the company. They also felt the number of stakeholders in the mix was too high. There were several CROs, data management companies, analytics companies and submissions partners involved and it created a very complex ecosystem in a global trial execution. The end to end technology platform-based solution is not just a solution to improve the current state of development affairs—it helps in creating solutions for the future as well. One such example is the virtual clinical trial.

When Pfizer experimented with the Research On Electronic Monitoring of OAB Treatment Experience in 2012, it gathered significant knowledge that would make the virtual trials a reality [13]. It is a technology platform which can educate potential trial participants through videos and contents, enroll subjects and investigators, and help distribute clinical supply materials to the subject's home. The investigators can upload test results and related information into the platform and enter relevant data in a standard format for better analytics and reports.

The whole trial can be done without creating huge trial sites with several trips for various stakeholders. The system can manage data in the format the sponsor wants and it creates real-time visibility of the trial status. This can have a clinical supply management module to create demand-supply status and risks in real-time to eliminate or reduce the huge clinical supply wastage.

MANUFACTURING

When you pick up a medicine from the pharmacy or any other store, you get it in a nice pack. You see a tablet or capsule strip inside or a bottle of liquid when you open the pack. You also see a product insert, the short document which lists all the product benefits, safety, risks, contact details in case of adverse events, etc. The product manufacturing and packaging of the product, making sure we as patients get the right product, happens in the manufacturing plant. This is the workhorse of a pharmaceutical company.

Pharmaceutical manufacturing follows a series of steps defined in the manufacturing process to produce medicines. This process is developed in the R&D, scaled up to the commercial manufacturing, approved by the FDA and other health authorities in a country before implementing them in a manufacture plant. The manufacturing process is static and every production batch needs to follow the process exactly the way it's defined and all the steps need to be completed. The process documentation for every production batch needs to be completed in real-time as various steps in the process are done—Good Manufacturing Practice (GMP) ensures documented evidence is completed during the operation and not as an after thought.

The pharmaceutical manufacturing process is divided into two main stages. The first one is known as Active Pharmaceutical Ingredient (API) manufacturing and the second one is "Formulations Development", the form we see in our medicine cabinet. The first stage is responsible for manufacturing the active drug component and the second stage uses this active drug and creates formulations using other non-drug material for effective binding, for release inside the body and for preserving it for longer. The final pharmaceutical products are available in various forms such as liquid, semi-solid and solid. The solid forms are capsules and tablets; semi-solids are creams, ointments, etc. and the liquid form includes solutions, gels, suspensions, emulsions and injectables. These medicines are ingested directly or used through medical devices.

Active Pharmaceutical Ingredients (API) or Bulk Drug Manufacturing Process

The description given in Figure 2.6 is a general view of the API manufacturing process. This is modified for a specific product which may not follow some steps whereas another product may use some extra steps.

The manufacturing process is driven by a production plan which is aligned with the demand plan provided by the sales team. The process starts with making all the equipment ready as per the GMP guidelines. There are two main process types used to manufacture pharmaceuticals—(1) chemical synthesis based on chemical reactions, and (2) bioprocessing based on the ability of microorganisms and cells to produce substances with medicinal values (fermentation technique). Chemical synthesis can be used to produce pharmaceutical products with relatively low molecular weights in large volumes in short time spans. In addition, various chemical modifications can be applied to enhance the activity of the substance produced, whereas the biopharmaceuticals are produced in a very controlled environment and need sophisticated technologies to successfully manufacture the right product. There are always chances of microbial contamination which can produce more impurity and toxic materials along with the desired product.

Chemical synthesis and the fermented product manufacturing process start differently. Chemical synthesis is carried out in reactors by adding various reactants in controlled environment, for example, temperature, pH, liquid concentration, etc. for reaction to take place. The fermentation process starts with sterilization of vessels, creating an environment where microbes can grow and produce the product. Most processes follow purification, crystallization and product filtration techniques to isolate products. The product is then dried in various drying conditions, milled to reduce crystal size or sifted to separate into various crystal sizes. Sev-

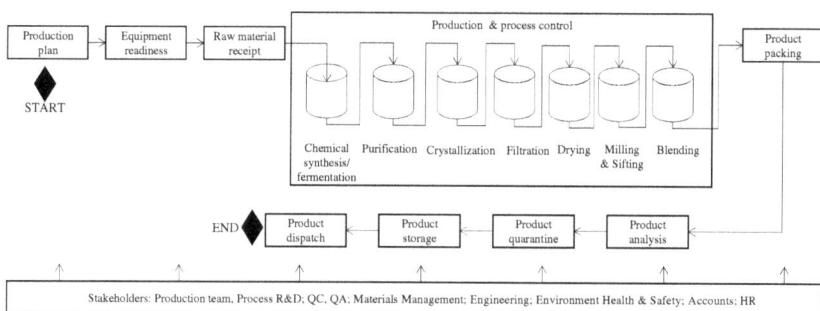

FIGURE 2.6   API manufacturing process.

eral batches at times are blended together for formulation process reasons. The blended product is packed as per the packing specification, and at times, it's packed to meet the order size. A quality control team takes samples of these packages for testing against pharmacopoeia specified tests. Packaged products are kept in quarantine until they are approved by quality control and certified in the packages. Certified products are moved into the finished product packaging area for shipping to customer locations.

In general, pharmaceutical plants produce many different products, and production lines must be kept separate from one another to prevent cross-contamination of products. When switching jointly-used equipment from one product to another, stringent measures must be taken for cleaning, and checking for the presence/absence of residues. In many cases, solvents and other combustible substances are used in addition to the raw materials, and this requires that the manufacturing plant buildings and facilities be fire-proofed, as well as other safety and security measures for highly flammable substances. Also, in some cases, corrosive fluids are used and equipment requires special linings or other protective measures.

Formulated Product Manufacturing Process

The API manufactured as described in the earlier section cannot be consumed by the patient. This needs to be formulated into various dosage forms suitable for consumption. Most pharmaceutical formulations follow a step by step approach as described in the approved manufacturing process (see Figure 2.7).

The manufacturing steps begin with the cleaning of the equipment and dispensing of raw materials as per the Bill of Material (BOM) in an area free from dust and other contaminants. The ingredients are blended in a blender. The blended product is then moved to a wet mill to reduce

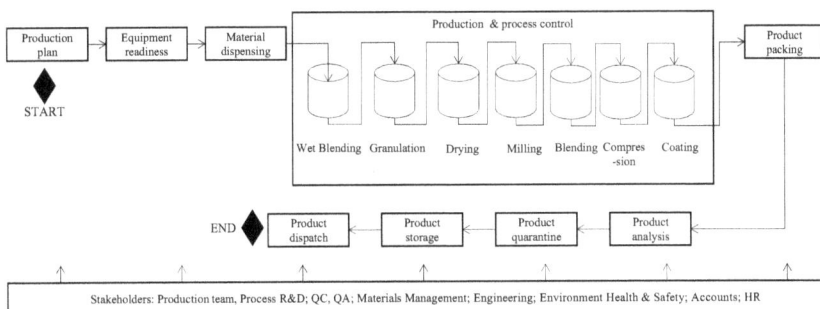

FIGURE 2.7 Formulation process.

the particle size of the mix. The milled product is then dried and taken for dry-blending and milling, and stored in sealed product drums. Quality control takes samples of granulation, and sometimes other intermediate products as defined in the Batch Manufacturing Record (BMR).

The granulation is compressed to make tablets by using a tablet press. This is done after the Quality Control (QC) approves the granules. The tablets are stored in drums and moved to the quarantine area for QC sampling. This is then moved for packaging operations after QC approval. The tablets are packaged by using various packaging techniques based on the product type. The packaged products are quarantined in the finished product quarantine area for QC sampling, analysis and release of the Certificate of Analysis (CoA). The product is ready to dispatch to the customer once the CoA is released.

The following unit operations are used in API or formulations manufacturing processes:

Chemical synthesis. This is the discipline in which various forms of bioactive compounds are synthesized or modified through chemical reactions. Chemical synthesis is a process in which a product or product combinations are formed through chemical reactions of ingredients added to the reaction vessel. In the pharmaceutical manufacturing context, this reaction needs to be reproducible, and should work every time to produce the same product or by-products. A chemical synthesis requires reagents or reactants mixed in a reaction vessel (reactor) in a controlled environment to establish reproducibility. The product output in a chemical synthesis is expressed by the "yield", which is the ratio of "weight of the product actually produced" to the "possible quantity theoretically produced".

Fermentation. Fermentation is a process for the production of a product by the mass culture of microorganisms. The growth of a microorganism may result in the production of a range of metabolites, but to produce a particular metabolite the desired organism must be grown under precise cultural conditions at a particular growth rate. This makes the fermentation process harder to control and produce a bioactive compound repetitively. The microorganism identified to produce a product is introduced into a nutrient medium in a controlled vessel (fermenter) that supports its growth and produces the desired product.

Purification. The technique is to separate a desired product from other by-products produced through chemical synthesis or fermentation processes. There are several purification techniques used in pharmaceutical manufacturing including filtration, solvent extraction, crystallization, centrifugation, evaporation and distillation.

Crystallization. Crystallization is the process of formation of solid crystals precipitating from a solution of a pharmaceutical product produced chemically or through fermentation. Crystallization is achieved by changing the solubility conditions of the solute by means of changing temperature, pH, etc. of the solution. The crystallization happens through nucleation and growth. The crystal form nucleates and then grows to the full crystal throughout the entire crystallization process. Crystallization is very process dependent and any changes from the protocol can either make the product amorphous, or crystal may entrap impurities from the solution.

Filtration. Filtration is a process in which the solid is separated from the liquid or gas. The commonly used mechanism is to use a filter material through which only one fluid can pass.

Drying. Drying is a process to remove water or solvents from the product that were used in the crystallization or filtration process. This process is often used as a final production step before packaging pharmaceutical products. A source of indirect heating to remove the vapor produced by the process is used. Vacuum drying is also used to optimize the drying process.

Milling. Milling is a process to break solid materials into smaller particles. This is typically done using mechanical forces. Grinding may serve the purposes of increasing the surface area of a solid, manufacturing of a solid with a desired grain size and pulping of resources.

Sifting. The sifting or sieving process separates material with various particle sizes. Pharmaceutical products at times are packaged using a very specific particle size as that is needed for tablet or capsule manufacturing. The sieving technique separates a specific size of particle from the rest.

Blending. Blending is a unit operation which makes heterogeneous material more homogeneous or coats one product with another.

Granulation. Granulation is a process to increase particle size, in a way the reverse of the milling operation. Granulation can be a wet granulation where solvents are used to help the process. In case of a heat- or moisture-sensitive product the granulation is done in dry conditions.

Compaction. The compaction process is used to reduce the size of the powdery product into a solid tablet. Normally powered by hydraulics, compactors take many shapes and sizes.

Packaging. Packaging is the technique of enclosing products. Packaging and containment help to protect the product, reduce damage, make transportation convenient and give marketing benefits.

Manufacturing Teams

Various units come together at a manufacturing plant to make a product: the Production Unit, Quality Control, Process R&D, Materials Management, Engineering Maintenance, HR, Finance, and Environment Health & Safety. While the manufacturing shop-floor personnel manage the end to end process and unit operations to produce a quality product, all the other units support them to make this happen.

The **Production Unit** consists of the production manager, supervisor, chemists and unit operations teams. The production team carries out the production activities as per the predefined manufacturing process. The major documents they follow or create during running a batch are the following: batch manufacturing record, raw material issue record, inventory of finished product, intermediates, in-process materials and raw materials in the plant, process validation record, cleaning record, equipment utilization chart, production record, daily operations report, shift log record, Standard Operating Procedure (SOP), Material Safety Data Sheet (MSDS), production plan, maintenance plan, personnel training records, etc. These documents are needed as per the good manufacturing practice (GMP) and are auditable by health authorities, e.g. US FDA, EMA, JMHLW, TGA, etc.

Several information technology products are used today to ensure compliance to the end to end production process as per the approved production process—Manufacturing Execution System (MES) is one such system. The product inventory and distribution mechanism is easily managed using various Enterprise Resource Planning (ERP) products such as SAP or Oracle. If trained properly these technologies are easy to use, help to execute steps better, keep records of all activities and easily produce documented evidence during audits. Several document management systems are available that are specifically designed for the pharmaceutical industry with full compliance with FDA guidelines including computer system validation and 21 CFR Part 11 compliance as appropriate.

The key responsibility of the **Quality Control** unit is to ensure a quality product is produced and distributed for use. This requires ensuring quality at every stage of the production—the raw material, in-process material, packaging material and the finished product. Quality control becomes overwhelming at times from the sheer volume of activities and it becomes unreasonable to test each and every sample in the manufacturing process. Instead they draw samples as per the statistical process of sampling, which ensures a limited number of samples representing the entire size of the material under test. Another key aspect of the quality control is to track product stability data. Quality control keep a control sample to establish the stability of the product and take actions, including product recall, if desired product stability is not found in an accelerated stability study. In this process the product is exposed to the simulated adverse conditions to check their quality status and performance for a period of time. They produce several records for a product including a list of the raw material, the finished product, material specification, in-process check details and result, product distribution list, product stability data, product control sample record, product impurity profile, product analysis protocol, analysis result, reagent lists, reagent preparation methods, self-inspection record, microbial analysis of product and utilities, analytical instrument list, instrument calibration record, analytical method validation records, SOP, MSDS and training records.

While many quality control labs prefer to run their operations manually, there are many good technology systems available today to make the operation smarter. There are several software products to manage lab execution and documentation such as the Lab Information Management System (LIMS), Electronic Lab Notebook (eLN), Quality Management Systems (QMS) and Document Management Systems (DMS). The Irish Department of Agriculture has connected all its laboratories in Ireland to reduce documentation errors by 80% and increase information sharing between labs significantly. This connected system even integrates with the SAP system to track the material flow seamlessly [14]. Close to 50% of pharmaceutical laboratories today use at least one lab system to manage operations or data. There is huge potential for the industry to increase technology usage and create a paperless lab environment to reap the automation benefits to increase productivity, reduce non-compliance, increase knowledge share and of course reduce cost significantly. Several pharmaceutical companies have embarked on this initiative [15].

The **Quality Assurance** unit provides assurance to the company and its customers of establishing a quality operation and consistent performance of producing quality products. This team develops a quality system in the plant and ensures proper implementation. The quality system consists of the quality of facility, process, people, equipment and technologies in a manufacturing facility. The team looks at operational data for quality and creates continuous improvement plans. The quality assurance team is responsible for tracking of customer complaints and investigates the matter to closure. The major documents maintained in this unit are the following: master manufacturing process, batch manufacturing record review report, product rejection record, customer complaints review, deviation investigation, product quality trends, product yield consistency analysis, product traceability analysis, stability data review, internal quality audits, product distribution record review, process validation planning, equipment qualification planning, system validation planning, regulatory submission planning, preparation of dossier, self-inspection record, customer complaints record and closure report, SOP, personnel training records and more.

The **Process R&D** which is connected with a manufacturing unit is responsible for manufacturing process improvement and process trouble-shooting at the plant. They research batch data, product quality issues, yield improvement and safety improvement on a continuous basis. This unit creates and uses several documents including the laboratory notebook, literature survey record, lab experiments details, lab trial batch record, process development report, lab chemical inventory, SOP, MSDS and training documents. Technology information and data sources with trend reports are a very useful system for the Process R&D team.

The **Materials** department receives, stores and issues raw material to the plant after dispensing to the size of a manufacturing batch. The important activity is also to segregate materials as per their properties, uses or any other regulatory requirements. The entire warehouse needs to be segregated as per the predefined areas for storage of different materials. There should be distinct separation between raw material, finished product, packing material, under test material, rejected material and approved material. Storage areas need to be clean and monitored for temperature, dust control and humidity levels if the storage condition specifies the limits for specific products. This unit may also be responsible for shipping materials to customers as per the orders received and also to record any customer complaints related to product distribution and packaging issues. There are several activities and documented evidence created in this unit—raw material list, finished product list, packing material list, inventory of raw material, finished product, quarantined material, rejected material and packing material, approved vendor list, goods receipt notes, material issue record, environment monitoring record, SOP, MSDS, CoA, customer complaints and training records.

The **Engineering** and **Maintenance** teams are responsible for two major activities—the plant equipment maintenance and producing utilities to run the plant. These activities are very distinctive and at times handled by separate teams but can be combined under the same umbrella for synergies. The maintenance activities include various engineering services including mechanical, electrical, civil and instrumentation. All the equipments used in the process need to be qualified for the purpose and need to be maintained qualified always for consistent performance. The utility division handles production of HVAC including steam, compressed air, nitrogen, hot water, cool water, chilling system, vacuum, etc. needed to manufacture products, store or ship as per the condition specified in the process. They need to maintain similar documents described in the production section including equipment master (name, specification, MOC, location, purchase history, etc.), equipment qualification (DQ, IQ, OQ, PQ), plant layout details, Planned Preventive Maintenance (PPM), instrument calibration, inspection records such as boiler, weights and measures, plant insurance, electrical, environmental protection agency, engineering drawings, computer system validation, utility generation details (quality, generation, uses, loss, etc.), solvent storage facilities, SOP and training documents.

Environment Health and Safety ensures safety, health and environmental conditions in the manufacturing unit. This includes people, plant, machinery and the whole environment, not only the plant area but also the adjacent areas. This team analyses the process for safety, effect on the environment, health hazard to the personnel working nearby and the effect on the larger society. The following documentation are important for this team—HAZOP (Hazard & Operability) study of process and plant, area classification data, safety permit system, safety equipment monitoring, Material Safety Data Sheet (MSDS), environment protection device functionality, effluent treatment facilities, water balance record, COD (Chemical Oxygen Demand), BOD (Biological Oxygen Demand) trends, accident reports, incident studies, meteorological data, SOP and training records.

The **Human Resources** team at a manufacturing plant ensures hiring and retaining the right skills, and provides proper training to personnel to gain and improve skills needed to carry out their jobs. This team maintains the hygienic condition in the manufacturing area and monitors employees' health on a regular basis. The team ensures role-based organization structure, qualification of various roles, job description of roles, training plan and execution, personnel hygiene policy, policy for hygienic work conditions, employee signature album and SOP.

The **Accounts** team continuously monitors the batch output, in-process material, yield trends and determines the product cost. This analysis shows production efficiency and scope for reducing production cost. Various records kept by this team are for product cost trends, utility cost trends, overhead cost trends, product yield trends and SOP.

Technology-Driven Improvement Opportunities

When I advised a large pharmaceutical manufacturing set-up in Illinois, USA, to increase their speed of product release, I found an astonishing technology solution to make it happen sooner and better. This was almost a decade ago when the use of technology in a pharmaceutical plant was still in its infancy. But a group of open-minded executives from the shop-floor operations, QA, QC, distribution teams and operations management teams decided to bring in an IT-enabled solution to speed up the process. We connected plant instruments, implemented electronic workflow-based software to execute various process steps, introduced deviation flags automatically based on the pre-set criteria and managed batch records and batch analysis reports through a central document management library. This helped the QC Manager to receive all the information needed to make a release decision and release CoA in one fifth of pre-technology time.

A similar solution to improve CAPA (Corrective And Preventive Action) management in a manufacturing site was a huge success (see Figure 2.8).

This custom-developed IT solution helped to identify CAPA incidents, a step by step approach to investigations, remediation plan and incident closure in the manufacturing plant. The system had separate CAPA components for R&D and manufacturing to keep the two stakeholder groups separate. The system is designed to get data from existing IT applications and also provided manual data entry options for non-integrated interfaces. It had a deviation monitoring component to send alerts to concerned stakeholders and end to end CAPA workflow for tracking the entire remediation process. The technology has improved

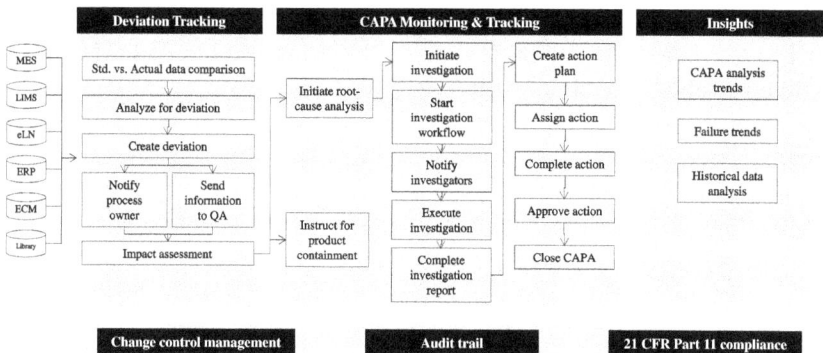

FIGURE 2.8   Deviation and CAPA management.

the QC productivity of the plant by 200% and made them 100% compliant in the FDA audits.

SUPPLY CHAIN MANAGEMENT

The definition of the supply chain is not uniform. Many describe this as a purchasing and procurement function; some describe it as warehousing, distribution and transportation. It also gets defined as the sourcing of capital and labor. The Council of Supply Chain Management Professionals combines some of these elements to describe this as "planning and management of all activities involved in sourcing, procurement, conversion and logistics management activities. This includes coordination and collaboration with channel partners—suppliers, intermediaries, third-party service providers, and customers. So the supply chain management integrates supply and demand management within and outside a company" [16].

Supply chain management is an approach to integrate suppliers, manufacturers, warehouses and stores. This function effectively forecasts, distributes, tracks and manages product storage, distribution and return to the right locations. The core components in the supply chain management are plan, source, produce, deliver and return. The supply chain demand-supply cycle is described in the diagram in Figure 2.9: supplier to customer loop.

Fundamentally, the supply chain management has the following broader components:

- *Customer demand management:* The demand management process creates the balance between customer requirements with the manufacturer's supply capabilities. The demand forecast is synchronized with the production, procurement, and distribution functions. The process

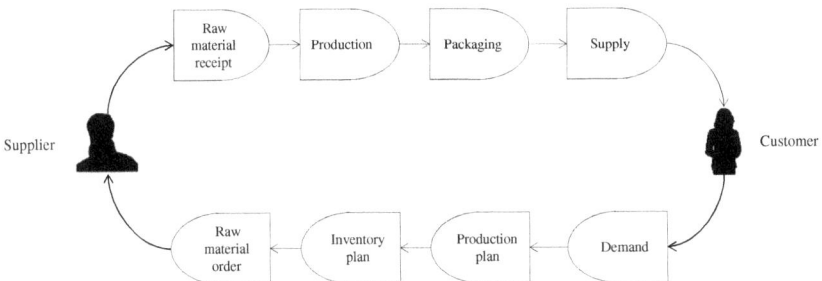

FIGURE 2.9 Demand-supply cycle.

also ensures the availability of contingency plans in the case of manu-facturing production issues. Systems such as CPFR (Collaborative Planning, Forecasting And Replenishment) or VMI (Vendor Managed Inventory) are widely used to manage the information.

- *Order fulfillment:* Order fulfillment is fundamental to an effective supply chain management. This can be achieved by creating an inte-grated operation between production, logistics and marketing plans. The right order visibility, collaboration between teams and effective contingencies can make the order fulfillment work better.
- *Manufacturing logistics:* Manufacturing logistics is the planning and coordination needed for product manufacturing. The production planning, scheduling and control of all activities have direct impact on the product movement and inventory which in turn impacts on the product supply to the customer.
- *Purchasing and supplies management:* The manufacturing logistics plan controls the purchasing of raw materials. These raw materials are arranged based on the production schedule, production batch size and usage of productions lines. The production schedule is always synchronized with the orders.
- *Distribution management:* Manufacturing companies work with various distribution companies to supply the product to its customers. The distribution design is an important aspect to decide on the chan-nels to be used for the product distribution. Some of the pharmaceut-ical products need special weather conditioning during distribution for their temperature sensitivity. This conditioning is applied to the product warehouse and operations management as well.
- *Returns management:* The returns management is not only a key aspect in the supply chain cycle, it also indicates the company's productivity status. An effective returns management can contribute significantly to the manufacturers' production efficiency.

One goal that is met through the supply chain is to balance the supply side with the demand. While the material flows from the manufacturer to the customer, the money and information flow back from the customer to the manufacturer. The right balance makes the manufacturer profitable.

Currently, two major industry situations are driving supply chain leaders to think outside the box. They are looking for technology-driven solutions. The first one is the impending ePedigree law to fight the prod-uct counterfeit problem. Pharmaceutical manufacturers need to comply with this for their 50% of the product portfolio by 2015 and for what remains by 2016. The wholesalers and re-packagers will need to comply by 2016 and the pharmacies and their warehouses need to comply by 2017. The requirement is very simple—the entire product needs to be tracked from manufacturing to the patient's shelf through a specific but indefinable number. The Food & Drug Administration (FDA) estimates that counterfeit drugs account for 10% of all medication in the US, while the EU believes between 1% and 3% of medicines sold across its member countries are fake. Clearly, these numbers endanger not only public health but also damage the global pharmaceutical industry. A robust supply chain backed by technology will eliminate this problem soon.

February 2010 was a dark month for the US pharmaceutical market. There was the astonishing theft of USD 75 million worth of antidepressants from the Eli Lilly distribution warehouse in Connecticut. There were two other thefts in the same month to increase the total amount stolen to about USD 200 million. The ePedigree law became even more relevant after these incidents.

With the ePedigree a product record is stored in an electronic form which contains information regarding the product and all the resulting transactions due to the change of ownership of a given product. Several technology solutions are used to track the product during manufacturing, during packaging, in the pallet, distribution packing and later to the wholesalers and retailers. The data generated at the various stages of the product movement gets stored in ERP systems for a pharmaceutical manufacturer.

The other major industry supply chain challenge is the clinical supply management. Today a big pharmaceutical company fails to use clinical supplies effectively which resulted in incinerating products worth tens of millions of dollars every year. This significantly adds to the product development cost.

Interestingly, a technology-enabled end to end supply chain management solution can reduce this product wastage significantly. I have experienced development of customized ERP solutions for clinical supplies at large pharmaceutical and CRO organizations. This solution provides an integrated solution for product packaging, label management, order management, planning and forecasting, distribution, warehouse management, expiry tracking, data management and analytics.

The packing module differs from the standard product packaging as it varies based on the clinical trial type—open blind, single blind or double blind. The packaging also depends on product randomization. Randomization is a process to allocate medication, either using the active product or a placebo, based on a predefined ratio in the trial protocol. Clinical sample packages need to match the desired product in a trial group at a site for the most efficient utilization. Verification tools are used to ensure the right components are used for primary and secondary packaging as per the randomization. It is important for blinded study to make sure randomization logic is followed during the packing in the warehouse.

Specific labels are printed to match the sample needed by a trial type and distribution. The primary labels are to indicate the sample and secondary labels to identify a specific consignment based on a site need. The labels are created as per the trial protocol.

A process order needs to be managed very effectively. As clinical trial products come with a very short shelf-life, this needs to be produced, distributed and used within a very short cycle time. The traditional order management and distribution very often fail to meet this requirement.

The demand management and planning of clinical supplies are maintained based on supply forecast characteristics. Forecast characteristics include geographical location, trial parameters including treatment group, pack types, dosing schedule and the enrolment data.

The distribution of clinical supplies has significant improvement opportunities and is a critical part of making supply management much more efficient. The distribution is a bit complex as it involves several internal and external agencies. The manufacturer, distributor, transporter depot, site level storage and distribution to the labs—all need to be tracked and supplied as per the trial plan. Over or under supply is not an acceptable solution at all.

The warehouse management ensures the right product receipt, inspection and storage as per the trial packaging needs for speedy delivery to the sites. Clinical trial goods are stored based on categorization—safe segregation of materials by hazard classification, traceability of material and batches to location and bin level, storage at the correct temperature range.

The most important aspect is the effective master data management, tracking data and analytics to improve supply chain visibility. Which product is needed where and when is the foundational element to reduce clinical supply wastage. Effective use of technology has helped improve the visibility significantly at several pharmaceutical and CRO organizations.

MARKETING

As Peter Drucker described, "marketing is the whole business seen from the point of view of its final result, that is, from the customers' point of view". When you watch the TV ad of a medicine only for a few seconds it may or may not last too long in your mind. If it has, the marketing team of the manufacturing company is successful, otherwise the team has failed. We are speaking about the team who is responsible for spreading the word of a company's products and services to the world. The marketing function is responsible for influencing non-purchasers to buy their product or service.

Currently, sales and marketing teams in pharmaceutical companies are often brand focused and work largely in brand, geographical and customer silos. This means that customer facing teams, such as field sales, brand management, and medical affairs, interact with customers separately without adequate communication or co-ordination. Under such circumstances, pharmaceutical companies fail to present a unified face and value proposition to their customers.

It is clear that a brand, field force-centric model that relies primarily on a large field sales force is ineffective in tackling these challenges and delivering the required revenue results. This chapter navigates through some of these challenges and describes the new model pharmaceutical companies that are adapting to combat them. The key role for marketing organizations is to monitor external and internal factors that can impact on a company's growth, margin and compliance and create product massaging. They develop marketing content to suit the channels that would work better for a brand in a specific location. The channel mix consists of face-to-face, web, email, mail, video, remote video, self-detail and more.

Shifting Marketing Dynamics

There are many factors that drive the need for a fundamental change in the pharmaceutical marketing model, including evolving consumer behavior and expectations, reinforced regulations, change in physician preferences, and a need for increased transparency at all levels of operation. Some of the following factors prompt this marketing model transformation:

> *Revenue pressures:* With an increasing number of branded drugs coming off patent, pharmaceutical companies are faced with a sharp reduction in sales revenue that is unlikely to be compensated by new brands. All operational costs are under great scrutiny as companies brace for lower revenues
>
> *Low field force effectiveness:* Pharmaceutical representatives are unable to get quality face-time with physicians. Physician's "do not call"

list is ever-increasing to make face-to-face detailing less likely. Thus, pharmaceutical companies do not earn an adequate return on their significant investment in field force

Increasing payer control: Payers are taking greater control over treatment choices with safety, efficacy and cost as their key priorities. Pay for performance is an emerging trend that is gaining momentum across various countries

Patient awareness: The pervasiveness of the internet, as well as growing awareness of healthcare, product, nutrition and lifestyle choices have created a more informed breed of patients

Economic and healthcare reform/regulatory climate: The recent economic crisis, impending healthcare reform and continued concerns regarding drug efficacy and safety will keep up the pressure on all aspects of the pharmaceutical business.

As a result of pharmaceutical companies responding to these industry dynamics, a new marketing model is emerging. While it is difficult to predict how exactly this change will unfold, some fundamental principles are becoming clearer:

Expansion of the Definition of "Customer"

For years, pharmaceutical companies have regarded the physician as their primary customer. However, recently the physician's hold on the prescription decision has slackened, as payer control, Pharmacy Benefit Management (PBM) influence and patient knowledge have grown. There are many key influencers in the purchasing decision, including hospitals, key opinion leaders, university medical centers and other specialized organizations. The pharmaceutical marketing model needs to be aware that one solution does not fit all and tailored approaches are required for each demographic.

Exploitation of New Channels of Communication

Customers are increasingly using the internet to research product information on their own, as they need it, whenever they need it. The positive outcome to this is an increase in reactive sales from online engagement. However, this can't be relied on and pharmaceutical companies need to reach a balance between face-to-face interaction and online delivery of content. Pharmaceutical companies will need to account for this changing trend and be proactive about investing in digital content that can be delivered through multiple communication channels. If done right, this can help pharmaceutical companies reduce their sales and marketing cost significantly while improving the effectiveness of the physician/customer interaction.

Targeted Messaging

As pharmaceutical marketing teams refine their customer messaging, they must focus on messages specific to a customer need in a given customer segment. Though customer analysis already takes place, there needs to be a significant increase in the collection of customer data, understanding of customer needs, and an increased ability to respond in a personalized manner.

From a sales interaction standpoint, the ability of the pharmaceutical company to respond to a customer query through the customer's preferred communication channel, with pertinent information, will dramatically improve the quality of the interaction. Collations of these inputs should form a critical input to the marketing plan.

Higher Emphasis on Patient Wellness

Today many patients are very well informed about personal health and spend considerable time researching disease conditions and available treatment options. Many benefit from support groups, especially where there is a need for lifestyle change or long-term care. As pharmaceutical companies focus on patient education and motivation, they should also look for opportunities to reinforce compliance with prescription regimes and behavior modification, as appropriate within regulatory boundaries. Social networking sites provide a great platform to motivate internet savvy patients at a very low cost of individual interaction.

The growing interest in "pay for performance" reinforces the focus on patient wellness and taking a holistic view of the treatment. Going forward, pharmaceutical companies must focus on the safety, benefits, cost-effectiveness and personalization of products to remain competitive and secure payment for their product.

So pharmaceutical marketing needs to move into an emerging model which will result in significant benefits for customers, as well as for the company. There are significant benefits for customers to have access to, and control over the information, improved outcomes and accessibility of the pharmaceutical company. Pharmaceutical companies can gain significant financial value, as well as improvement in sales and marketing outcomes from the investment to move to the new model. The model will encourage an increase in revenue from new prescriptions, better patient adherence, and customer loyalty despite the availability of generic products. There will also be a cost saving for the marketing teams, as fewer resources will be needed to support the field force operations. In the long term, there will be improvement of overall healthcare benefits and cost as the patients get more options for their wellness than treatment of diseases.

How Will a Marketing Team Set the Direction for Change?

Moving to a new marketing model represents a significant transformation. The first step is to establish the case for change and securing senior management buy-in. The other steps are to:

- Establish a robust business case for how value will be created for customers and for the company, and at what cost
- Define the business capabilities underpinning the realization of value
- Define the implications on sales and marketing processes; for example, what is the impact on the organization, is there a need for new technology, what will be the data requirements, etc.
- Identify appropriate change management and communication steps to ensure adoption and accountability of the new model
- Making strategic choices on prioritization and sequencing to result in a practical implementation roadmap.

Design the Details—Embedding Value into the New Model

The next step is to ensure that the estimated value can be delivered through the marketing model. There are choices to be made in leveraging a pharmaceutical company's existing capabilities and assets, and what new capabilities will be needed to build this from scratch. Key elements across the sales and marketing model are described in the Figure 2.10.

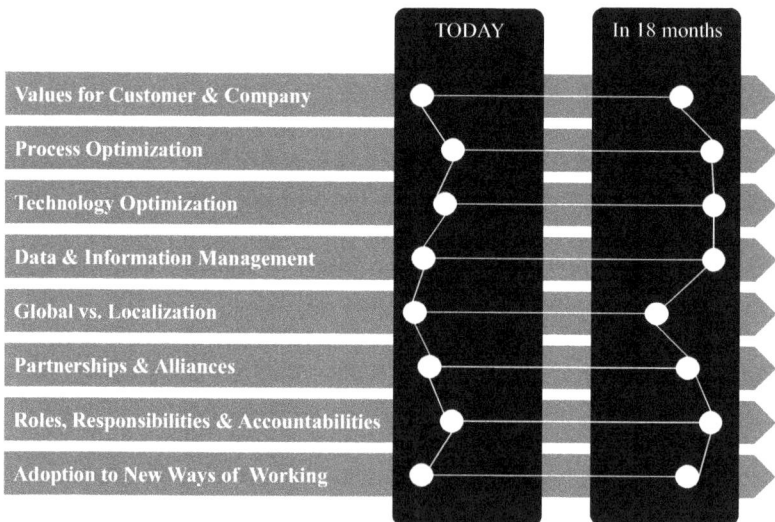

FIGURE 2.10 Marketing value benchmarking model.

Making it Happen—Ensuring Adoption and Realizing Value

A change of higher magnitude has many moving parts that need to be synchronized for successful value realization. These encompass multiple functional elements in marketing and different aspects including people, data, technology and process.

Some recurring themes that help to make a new model work better are:

- Customer first: Keeping the customer at the forefront of all decisions and taking an outside-in perspective to the program
- Stakeholder adoption and accountability: Ensuring adoption and accountability across the key stakeholders. There is a need to address this through clear and consistent messaging as well as deliberate change management activities. For example, it is very important that physicians/customers look at this as a value-added interaction instead of a sales push
- Technology choices and execution: Making the right technology choices, leverage of existing assets, as well as flawless execution need an upfront strategy. As one enters into this space, they should consciously look to leverage a third party platform and service offerings wherever these exist. This can help to get to market faster, bring capabilities that have been honed by early adopters such as retail, consumer product goods, and minimize the risk/investments to keep the platforms current
- Data quality and governance: Recognizing that the importance of good data is central to success in the new model, good quality data about physicians, touch points, prescription behavior, preferences, etc. are vital to delivering personalized messages to the right target segment. Refining this on a continuous basis and establishing the 360 degree feedback loop will also need data about activities/events and outcomes/behavior. The usage of marketing content through the constant source of market data would help refine the content. As too much data quickly creates an overload and becomes unusable, a robust governance to design standards and monitoring execution at all levels would make the strategy work.
- Incremental business value delivery: Like all programs, it is important to bring early momentum by delivering value incrementally to the key stakeholders. The marketing shift is a multi-year journey but internal and external stakeholders need to see tangible benefits starting in the first year.

Pharmaceutical companies' marketing models need to be evaluated as the external world has changed significantly. The change in customer demand, competition behavior, globalization and shift of business to emerging markets have put substantial pressure on marketing organization and this needs to be handled by adopting a new model.

SALES

While marketing establishes a product strategy, product messaging and a sales plan across various geographies, the field sales teams take over locally to execute the selling process.

A sale is the process in which a buyer and the seller discuss a product or service which is needed by the buyer. The seller tries to convince the buyer of the suitability of the product to make the sale. Communication can happen in many different ways including a face-to-face meeting, using audio/video or sending marketing materials to the buyer. This process has undergone significant changes recently due to the advancement of digital and mobile technologies. While the work can be done using many different methods, the fundamental sales steps are similar across various sales types.

Customer and Prospect Profiling

This is all about knowing your prospect or customer based on their buying pattern, buying history and previous call details. The Sales Manager initiates the sales planning process. A sales planning process is specified in detail at a territory planning level with specific assignments to the sales teams.

Prospecting is a very important activity for the sales team. This involves identification of a potential buyer, qualifying them and converting them to a lead who will very likely buy the product or service.

Sales Call Planning

Once customer profiling is done the sales team needs to segment the customers (for the sake of simplicity I will not specify prospects separately) and create a call plan. This plan would include reviewing customer data, reviewing earlier call results, if any, defining call objectives and planning the presentation.

Deliver the Message

On average during a visit to the physician's office, a sales representative gets less than a minute to give the physician the details of their product safety, benefit, risk factors, etc. The marketing message needs to be razor sharp, extremely concise and the sales person needs to deliver it flawlessly within the minute that they have. This is quite a difficult job without the right marketing support and extensive training.

Call Review and Record

The sales representative should record all calls to various prospects and customers. This information will be used for call analysis and to customize marketing messaging based on how well the call went with the customer. If the call was for a prospect and the sales person indicates the possibility of a sale, this prospect moves to the "lead" category. The lead will then be followed up with specific marketing material which may help close the sale. So, every call is important to the organization and the sales person should record the call in detail.

Sales Management Reports

This includes actual sales, sales pipeline, times and expenses report and activity report. These are required not only for plan refinement or internal management purposes but for regulatory reasons as well. Sales activities and expenses are monitored by the health authorities to ensure they do not promote off-label sales and do not influence customers by giving gifts or any other monetary means. The US Sunshine Act is specifically designed to monitor sales spend and all the companies are required to report this annually.

Sample Management

The Prescription Drug Marketing Act (PDMA) requires pharmaceutical manufacturers to have policies, procedures, and proper training to distribute product samples. An end to end tracking of all samples should be maintained to ensure a sample is used for its intended purposes only. The sales representative carries this huge compliance requirement while distributing samples to the physicians. They need to record samples and take the physician's signature as the documented evidence of distribution of samples.

There are several technology solutions to manage samples. This IT solution is integrated with the customer relationship management (CRM) system to connect a physician to a sales representative's call. The system also records any order of samples by a physician. This order is processed through the sample distribution system and delivers samples to the physician. This user-friendly system has the capability of capturing the physician's signature electronically. It also ensures tracking of sample requests and evidence of distribution, inventory management and reconciliation processes, captures any process deviations, and reporting can be done using a single system.

Scheduling

The sales management function has a huge responsibility to keep a company's stake high in the market by constantly increasing the revenue growth. A Regional Manager expects that a sales person will call on several physicians and pharmacies each day. In addition to that a sales person also needs to organize symposia every month or two. While working on a sales management process improvement project, I saw the daily schedule of a sales person from 8 am to 9 pm—it starts with a breakfast meeting with a physician and ends with a dinner with another physician or a pharmacist. The sales representative also needs to undergo training, attend a couple of seminars and organize video detailing at a time suitable for the physician, etc. All of these tasks have to be accomplished while ensuring weekly administration and regulatory tasks are done on time. There is much more to this job than just calling on doctors to prescribe your brand. A successful sales person is very methodical, drives business through proper planning process, reviews accomplishments periodically and fine-tunes the plan as needed. This is indeed a role of multi-tasking and there's no scope for making mistakes even in a high pressure situation.

Incentive and Compensation Management

An incentive program is a formal way to evaluate sales performance and reward sales personnel. The rewards could be in the form of promotion or increased pay or any other form of recognition. Incentive programs are particularly used to motivate employees, attract new talents, develop them and retain them.

Travel and Expenses (T&E)

Travel and expenses must be reported in the defined format as this is not only used for tracking expenses, it also gets audited by the regulatory authorities. These reports include a travel schedule, call details, and expenses details—expenses on customers are specifically scrutinized as it's a regulated item. Some T&E examples are travel, customer entertainment, office expenses, promotional content, electronics and mileage allowances.

John, a friend of mine, called me late on a December evening while I was at the Phillies stadium watching a Mets & Phillies baseball game. John is a Vice-President of a mid-sized pharmaceutical company and manages the sales team in the US. He wanted me to meet with his regulatory VP very urgently. Kelly, their regulatory VP, John and I met in that week to discuss their need for submitting the State Aggregate Spend and Transparency Report. Kelly managed the submission through a consulting company for the previous year but now she had a bigger problem to solve. The company had got bigger; hence John's sales team had become larger too. Their spend was much more and diverse. They had information in many different standard packages in a diverse set of technology systems. To top that, some data and systems came through a small company acquisition that year. Kelly and John wanted me to give them a solution to create and submit Aggregate Spend reports to six US states and also establish a long-term solution.

As part of the Patient Protection and Affordable Care Act, the USA has introduced The Sunshine Act to aggregate and monitor the total amount spent by healthcare manufacturers on individual Healthcare Professionals and organizations through payments, gifts, honoraria, travel and other means [17]. This initiative is a growing body of federal and state legislators that collectively address all or some of the following goals: (a) Provide transparency with regard to who, in the pharmaceutical industry, is contributing what benefits to which physician; (b) Mandate statutory reports at least once a year; and (c) Limit spend per physician. "Aggregate Spend" is the total, collective, cumulative amount spent by life sciences manufacturers (pharmaceutical, biotechnology and medical device organizations) on individual healthcare professionals and organizations through any means.

We looked at John and Kelly's organization and other key stakeholders to come up with a long-term solution. We also created a short-term agenda to create and submit state reports for that year as the long-term solution would take time to implement and would have delayed the submission.

The report needed to create a holistic picture of the company spend on HCPs. This should include all of their functions (the team structure may vary in other companies) as described below:

- Sales & Marketing
- R&D
- Medical Affairs
- Corporate Affairs
- External partners who manage meetings and conventions, etc.

The actual dataset was complex and at times duplicated in many systems or manually entered through a Microsoft spreadsheet. Manual reconciliation of data was essential for the company as they were using the end to end technology solution for the first time.

The dataset will become clearer as they start implementing the process and tools and all the stakeholders are fully trained on the new ways of managing spend on HCPs (see Figure 2.11). This aggregate state report needs the following information (only a subset):

Sales & Marketing
  • Meals, entertainment
  • Samples
  • KOL services fee
  • Patient education
  • Meetings and conventions
R&D Data Source
  • Trial execution
  • Liaisoning
  • Publication
3rd Party Vendors/Partners
  • Market research
  • Program management.

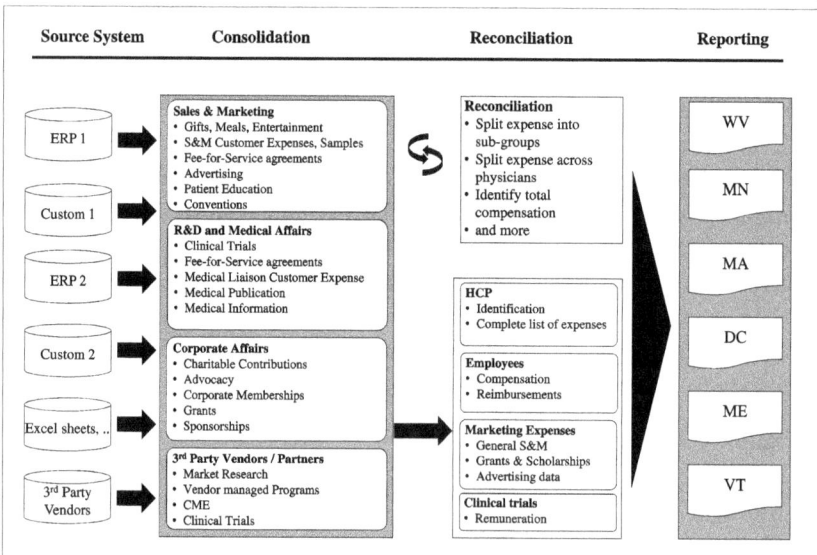

FIGURE 2.11   Sunshine Act functional landscape.

We had created an end to end process driven technology solution for Kelly. The core solution was a custom developed application with integration of many products (CRM, ERP, T&E, etc.). The reporting was done automatically using a standard reporting system. The solution did call for a significant people change management exercise. But, it was a success as their senior leaders were fully supportive to do the right thing in this fast growing pharmaceutical company. This was indeed a great success to improve business initiative using a technology solution. There are several such solutions to improve sales functions.

The sales team is the face of a pharmaceutical manufacturer to its customer base. They not only do the selling, they carry the company's reputation on their shoulder. They face several issues including product complaints, adverse events reports and customer relationship shortcomings. The sales team needs to record several of these inputs for their marketing and R&D teams to work on to improve brand messaging or improve product performance.

REGULATORY COMPLIANCE

A pharmaceutical company gets product marketing approval in a country through the drug approval process. In general, a drug approval process comprises various stages of applications submitted to the competent regulatory authority of the relevant country during the drug development life cycle. The drug discovery phase concludes with a regulatory submission, an IND (Investigational New Drug). The IND approval provides permission to conduct clinical trials on humans. If the drug continues to appear promising in the human trials, the pharmaceutical company submits the results to a regulatory authority in the form of an NDA (New Drug Application). The NDA is approved or rejected based on the documents and data to support product safety, efficacy and quality of the drug product. Companies apply for the Marketing Authorization of the drug by which they get the permission to sell and distribute the drug in a market. Safety monitoring of the drug continues in the form of Phase IV or post-marketing trials after the firm markets the drug. Health authorities continue monitoring the drugs in the market, which is known as Pharmacovigilance.

Worldwide Heath Authorities

Each country has its own health authority to provide regulatory guidelines for the manufacturing and marketing of products in the country.

The regulatory requirements for approval of a drug may differ from country to country.

The US Food & Drug Administration (FDA) is one such authority. The FDA is an agency of the United States Department of Health and Human Services, and is responsible for protecting and promoting public health. Their Code of Federal Regulation Title 21 (CFR 21) goes into great detail on considerations for the food and drug industry. The European Medicines Agency's (EMA) primary prerogative is to protect the health of humans and animals within the European Union through regulation of the medicines used by these populations. In the European Union a wide variety of regulatory procedures such as national, centralized, decentralized and mutual recognition are followed for approval of a new drug. The Therapeutic Goods Administration (TGA), a part of the Australian Government Department of Health and Ageing, is Australia's regulatory authority for pharmaceutical products and other therapeutic goods such as medical devices, blood products, vaccines, and topical sunscreen. Prior to marketing such a product in Australia, the TGA evaluates the product to ensure it has acceptable quality standards. In China the Drug Administrative Law authorizes the State Food & Drug Administration (SFDA) to approve new drugs for marketing.

At the highest level and across different countries the drug approval process predominantly consists of an application to conduct a clinical trial and application for marketing authorization. While the application information submitted is similar for all countries, the review process, rigor, time and fee may differ significantly. This also differs for product type. For example, the US FDA has a priority approval process for lifesaving drugs and an orphan drug approval process is faster than the normal approval process.

Pharma Compliance Regulations

Health authorities across countries have set certain compliance standards and regulations for pharmaceutical firms while they develop, manufacture and market their drug products. Compliance regulations ensure and enhance the safety of the consumers who use pharmaceutical products and companies are expected to strictly adhere to these compliance regulations. For the purpose of harmonization, the International Conference on Harmonization (ICH) has taken major steps for the harmonization of technical requirements for the registration of pharmaceuticals for human use. It's not a governmental entity, but plays a major role in the pharmaceutical industry on a global scale.

The ICH members consist of Europe, Japan and the United States. Their mission is to improve the efficiency of new drug development, testing, and registration, to reduce duplicative effort during clinical trials and harmonize the drug approval process across the globe. They do this by implementing harmonized guidelines and standards on quality, safety, and efficacy referred to as GxP guidelines where "X" stands for "Laboratory", "Clinical", "Manufacturing", etc. Good Laboratory Practice (GLP) is a set of quality guidelines initially developed by the FDA, but later adopted by the EPA (Environmental Protection Agency) and OECD (Organization for Economic Co-operation and Development). As such, GLP regulations provide guidelines on how a non-clinical health and environmental study should be planned, executed, documented, reported, and stored/archived.

All the pre-clinical studies are expected to comply with GLP guidelines. Additional details regarding the GLP principles published by the FDA can be found in 21 CFR Part 58 (Code of Federal Regulations Title 21, 2012). The ICH also publishes Good Clinical Practice (GCP) guidelines for investigators to conduct clinical trials in a way that protects the well-being of the human subjects, assures the safety and efficacy of the new drugs undergoing testing and the credibility of the results, and defines proper roles and responsibilities of the different actors during the clinical trial. These guidelines help investigators design, monitor, record, analyze and report clinical trials. The main objective is to set globally applicable standards for the conduct of clinical trials. Similar to GLP and GCP, Good Manufacturing Practices (GMP) are guidelines adopted by a variety of international regulatory agencies (including the FDA, Health Canada, TGA, WHO and the EU) to establish the right quality of products are made available for human and animal use.

Some of the major aspects of GMP include a high degree of control and validation around the manufacturing process, including any changes to the processes. Corrective And Preventive Action (CAPA) is one important aspect of GMP which focuses on investigation of errors and discrepancies and preventing their recurrence. Manufacturing procedures should be written in a clear and unambiguous manner, and records must be kept by operators and instruments as per Good Documentation Practices (GDP) to ensure traceability to the manufacturing batch. ICH also has created the Electronic Standards for the Transfer of Regulatory Information (ESTRI, E2B), the Common Technical Document (CTD and eCTD) used in regulatory submissions, and the Medical Dictionary for adverse event reporting and coding of clinical trial data (MedDRA). With greater reliance on technology to optimize processes, an increasing number of paper-based pharmaceutical records companies are shifting to electronic records; for that reason, the FDA has assembled guidelines as part of their Title 21 Code of Federal Regulations Part 11 (21 CFR Part 11). Any electronic records and signatures created and maintained by the pharmaceutical, biotech, and medical device industries for the purpose of FDA audits (including those created in the GCP, GLP, GMP settings) must comply with the Part 11 guidelines.

The complete electronic regulatory submission process demands that computer systems handle a huge amount of documents and related data and information. Proper functioning and performance of these systems play a vital role in consistency, reliability and credibility of the data. Therefore, the FDA has provided guidelines, known as Computer System Validation (CSV), for validation of accuracy of these systems. These guidelines provide the validation methods, requirement documentation, development and testing procedures, etc. to be followed to ensure the software is developed as needed and is fully functional as desired. Once the system is validated and certified, there are audits performed by the FDA for reviewing the performance and accuracy of the system over a regular interval of time.

Pharmaceutical companies invest a huge sum of money in drug development and therefore it is vital for them to make the drug a success in the market. Once they get Market Authorization approval, they move into the sales, marketing and promotional activities of the drug. These marketing activities of the drug product are regulated by different laws like the Sunshine Act, HIPPA, PhRMA, EFPIA, IFPMA, FFDCA, etc. The Sunshine Act is a US Law which makes it mandatory for pharmaceutical companies to compile and report their spendings (including "transfer of values" and payments) on individual doctors and physicians in hospitals to the Secretary of HSS in the specified format. Any manufacturer which operates in the US must comply with this law regardless of the manufacturing location. The purpose of this law is to break the financial relationship between drug/device manufacturers and the physician which results in an increase in treatment costs and influences the decision of which drug is to be included in the prescription.

In the US, the marketing of drug products must abide by the Federal Food, Drug, and Cosmetic Act (US FFDCA) and by the guidelines provided by Pharmaceutical Research and Manufacturers of America (PhRMA). These guidelines prohibit drug manufacturers from providing items of any value to healthcare providers including gift items, free samples, etc. In Europe, EFPIA (European Federation of Pharmaceutical Industries and Associations) ensures that pharmaceutical companies must conduct the promotion of the drug product in a truthful manner (so as to avoid deceptive practices and potential conflicts of interest between drug manufacturers and healthcare providers) and that product promotions must be in compliance with the law.

The International Federation of Pharmaceutical Manufacturers and Associations (IFPMA) is another such authority which looks after ethical promotion of drug products globally. There have been cases in which the Division of Drug Marketing have cited a few drug manufacturers violating FDA guidelines on disclosure of drug information over social media. Though FDA has published a draft, there are no guidelines by the FDA on the marketing of drug products online, so it is a challenge for pharmaceutical companies to meet the regulatory controls while utilizing the social media platform for product promotions and marketing.

Over time a strong nexus has been established between HCP and drug manufacturers. HCPs possess health information for their patients which can be of vital importance for drug manufacturers as it can be good information for clinical trials that can save both money and time for developing a drug. But this is a compromise of the patient information protection law. Therefore, in order to protect public health information from being used by a drug manufacturer or any other parties, Health Insurance Portability and Accountability Act (HIPAA) was put in place by the regulatory authorities. HIPAA protects the health information of individuals while simultaneously allowing the disclosure of health information which is required for the provision of quality healthcare.

Like other industries, pharmaceutical companies also have to abide by the Sarbanes Oxley Act (SoX) which enforces the accuracy of disclosed financial information. The main objective of SoX (originally known as The Corporate and Auditing Accountability, Responsibility and Transparency Act) is to prevent investors and other stakeholders from corporate and accounting scandals. This law enforces the CFO/CEO of the organization to individually certify the accuracy of financial information being disclosed to the public.

The diagram in Figure 2.12 shows the list of various regulations to be complied with for drug development, manufacture and marketing in various countries.

Current Industry Trends and Challenges

Pharmaceutical companies continue struggling with these stringent regulations, heavy penalties in case of non-compliance to regulations and adds time to already lengthy time to market. Companies are strug-

Discovery	Development	Manufacturing	Supply Chain	Sales & Marketing	IT
• Good laboratory practice • Good documentation practice • COMS guideline • CDER • CBER • Good labor practice • …and many more	• Good clinical practice • Good documentation practice • COMS guideline • CDER • CBER • HIPAA • …and many more	• Good manufacturing practice • Good documentation practice • GAMP5 • ISO9000 • OSHA • Weights & Measures • Boiler • Fire • SUPAC guideline • …and many more	• Good storage and shipping • Good documentation practice • Good distribution practice • Track and trace • ISO9000 • OSHA • Weights & Measures • Fire • …and many more	• PhRMA • OIG • Sunshine Act • False claims act • Good documentation practice • Good distribution practice • Education grants • Sample mgt • …and many more	• Computer system validation • 21 CFR Part 11 • GAMP5 • …and many more

FIGURE 2.12   Regulatory compliance examples.

gling to strike the right balance between regulation and innovation. Too much focus on compliance to regulations dilutes their focus on unstructured innovation for development and launch of a blockbuster drug to market. Less focus on compliance poses risks to patient safety, product quality, and even potential for misreporting financial data and ultimately heavy fines levied by the regulators.

To combat these challenges the industry, which has been notoriously resistant to IT in regulatory compliance space, is now showing an increased trend towards adoption of technologies including cloud computing, mobile devices, smartphones and social media to stay ahead of the competition.

Mobile devices and applications are fast becoming popular in the pharmaceutical industry. Merck have developed a smartphone application for the consumers of one of their drugs which is used for the treatment of allergies. This application needs to be installed on the consumer's smartphone and it captures the information about the customer location and subsequently provides the local pollen count of that area along with the details of the nearby medication facilities. With easy access to the pollen forecast for the current and following day, consumers get information and advice on dealing with their allergies [18]. This can potentially be improved by allowing consumers to report their allergy details but compliance issues around adverse events could make this complicated. The adverse events need to be recorded, investigated and reported to the health authorities. This currently prevents pharmaceutical companies from collecting user feedback in real-time.

The main aim pharmaceutical companies have is to improve the quality and efficiency of their operations. As companies are taking measures to implement new technologies to reduce their incidence of CAPA, studies are now estimating that 90% of drug manufacturing defects occur due to human error. Thus, pharmaceutical companies are employing techniques to reduce human error by addressing variables such as employee morale, sleep, incentives, and shifts, to name a few [19]. They are also implementing LEAN Six Sigma principles such as poka-yoke, where a process is "mistake proofed" by design, to ensure it is impossible for the error to occur. For a global pharmaceutical company, the primary challenge in addressing CAPA is to do it in a consistent and reliable manner across all sites worldwide. Bristol-Myers Squibb (BMS) has installed a CAPA solution which can interact with customers to respond to adverse events, product quality complaints and warnings from regulatory authorities, etc. This CAPA software allows the company to capture data and information about the errors and deviations and helps in developing corrective action plans [20]. This is a good example of the proper use of technology to improve a quality and compliance function.

There are several examples in the industry which use Enterprise Quality and Compliance (EQM) systems to reduce compliance issues significantly. Implementation of EQM has resulted in reduction in complaint resolution time by 78%, reduction in CAPA cycle time by 51% and reduction in deviation process cycle time by 72% [21].

FINANCE AND ACCOUNTS

While working in a plant or a lab you always find it hard to get your reagents or raw materials delivered quickly enough. There seems to be some hold-up somewhere in processing the order or the payment did not go through, etc. This happens because the company needs to keep the cash flow as per the financial plan. The cash flow is the balancing act between the sourcing of money and the spending of money. Money sources are sales, profits, reserves, loans, etc. and spend areas are the employee wages and salaries, expenses, insurance, raw material purchase, capital investments and other operating expenses. Finance and Accounts is responsible for handling the money for the entire organization.

An analysis of a company's financial position is essential to form an opinion and make a decision about a company's health. This information is vital for its employees, potential employees, investors, clients and the company's decision-makers to make any strategic decision. It is important to know if the current profitability is enough to maintain the costs of the capital.

A company accountant is a very specialized role and the person needs to be trained and certified. Company accountants are responsible for managing the finances, preparing and reporting financial performance, auditing financial statements, taking risks and forming a view or giving advice on investments. So, the accounting practice is broadly categorized into **financial**, **operational**, **auditing** and **advisory** areas.

Financial accounting is the fundamental task of the finance and accounting function. Financial transaction management in ledger is a major task; the accountants also ensure cash availability to run the business and thirdly, they make sure the company operates as per the financial guidebook and regulatory requirements. Major tasks include costing, accounts receivables, financial statements, financial ratios, payroll accounting, taxation and asset management.

The operational accountants are responsible for managing the financial condition of the business on a regular basis, e.g. monthly. This includes cash flow forecasting, budgeting, variance analysis, credits and collections, investor relations and competitor analysis.

The auditing and advisory accountants are responsible for financial auditing and investment advice respectively.

Finance and Accounts is responsible for preparing and reporting on the company's financial health position which is known as the Annual Report. This may change based on the relevant country's level of accounting policies but there are significant common elements. As an example, the US Securities and Exchange Commission (SEC) mandates that the annual report to be submitted as per the Form 10-K provides a comprehensive view of the company's business and financial health. The Form 10-K has four parts and 15 schedules:

Part 1: Description of Business, Risk Factor, Unresolved Staff Comments, Description of Properties, Legal Proceedings and Mine Safety Disclosures
Part 2: Market for Registrant's Common Equity, Related Stockholder Matters and Issuer Purchases of Equity Securities; Selected Financial Data; Management's Discussion and Analysis of Financial Condition and Results of Operations; Quantitative and Qualitative Disclosures About Market Risk; Financial Statements and Supplementary Data; Changes in and Disagreements With Accountants on Accounting and Financial Disclosure; Controls and Procedures; Other Information
Part 3: Directors, Executive Officers and Corporate Governance; Executive Compensation; Security Ownership of Certain Beneficial

Owners and Management and Related Stockholder Matters; Certain
Relationships and Related Transactions, and Director Independence;
Principal Accounting Fees and Services
Part 4: Exhibits, Financial Statement Schedules Signatures

The financial statement is the most common way to understand a company's financial situation in a summary view. The Profit and Loss (P&L) statement, Balance Sheet and Free Cash Flow (FCF) are the financial statements described below.

Profit and Loss (P&L) Statement

The P&L statement is the summary of revenue, costs to the revenue and expenses for a period, usually quarterly, half-yearly or yearly. This shows the topline (revenue) and bottom-line (profit) of the company for a period and it's a tool for the company to optimize their plans to improve topline and bottom-line.

A fully detailed P&L can be quite complex, but a simple one is described in Figure 2.13.

Profit & Loss Account		Q1	Q2
A	Net revenue	$ 200,000	$ 300,000
B	Cost of revenue	$ 130,000	$ 200,000
C=A-B	Gross profit	$ 70,000	$ 100,000
D	SG&A--sales, general & administrative expenses	$ 36,000	$ 75,000
E=C-D	Profit from operations	$ 34,000	$ 25,000
F	Other income	$ 2,000	$ -
G=E+F	Net profit before tax	$ 36,000	$ 25,000
H	Tax provision	$ 14,400	$ 21,600
I=G-H	Profit after tax	$ 21,600	$ 3,400

FIGURE 2.13   P&L example.

Balance Sheet

This statement in Figure 2.14 provides a balanced view of assets, liabilities and shareholder's equity in a defined period. This "snapshot" of the financial health shows what the company owns and owes and the shareholders' values. The term "balance sheet" balances the "source of finance" and "use of finance".

Balanced Sheet			
Asset		Liabilities	
Cash	$ 125,000	Accounts payable	$ 225,000
Accounts receivable	$ 175,000	Salary	$ 190,000
Short-term investment	$ 50,000	Interests	$ 50,000
Inventories	$ 75,000	Tax	$ 25,000
...		...	
Stock investment	$ 150,000	Long-term loan	$ 100,000
Property, equipment	$ 250,000	Provisions for liabilities and charges	$ 50,000
Intangable assets	$ 50,000	Shareholder's equity	$ 250,000
Total assets	$ 875,000	Total liabilities	$ 890,000

FIGURE 2.14 Balanced sheet.

Free Cash Flow (FCF)

The FCF indicates the cash movement in and out of the company in a given time period. This cash flow is available to take care of stakeholders including employees, equity holders, debt holders, and stock holders. A sample FCF form is shown in Figure 2.15.

While financial statements provide an excellent view on the company's financial situation, several trends help determine the true health of a company. There are several financial ratios where items are divided by one another to reveal their logical interrelationships, but the most important ones are given in Figure 2.16. These ratios can be created to compare companies, industries, or different time periods within one company.

	Net Free Cash Flow	
A	Income	$100,000
B	Depreciation	10,000
C	Accounts receivable	-3,0000
D	Inventory	-10,000
E	Expenses paid	5,000
F	Accounts payable	5,000
G	Accurals	-15,000
H=sum(A:G)	Operating cash flow	$65,000
I	Investments	10,000
J	Plants & equipments	-50,000
K=I+J	Long-term investment cash flow	-40,000
L	Loans	30,000
M	Dividend paid	-40,000
N=L+M	Finance activities cash flow	-10,000
O=H+K+N	Net increase in cash flows	$15,000

FIGURE 2.15 Net Free Cash Flow.

Ratio	How to calculate	Health indicator if ratio increases	Ratio	How to calculate	Health indicator if ratio increases
Current Ratio	Current assets/Current liabilities	Green	Inventory Turnover or stock turnover ratio	Annual cost of goods sold/Inventory	Red
Accounts Payable Turnover Ratio	Total supplier purchases/(Beginning accounts payable + Ending accounts payable) / 2	Red	Net Profit Ratio	(Net profit / Net sales) x 100	Green
Accounts Receivable Turnover Ratio	Net Annual Credit Sales/(Beginning Accounts Receivable + Ending Accounts Receivable) / 2	Green	Operating Ratio	(Production expenses + Administrative expenses)/Net sales	Red
Cash Ratio	(Cash + Cash equivalents)/Current liabilities	Green	Price Earnings Ratio	Current market price per share/Earnings per share	Red
Debt to Equity Ratio (Gearing ratio)	(Long-term debt + Short-term debt + Leases)/Equity	Red	Acid test ratio	(Cash + Marketable securities + Accounts receivable)/Current liabilities	Green
Dividend Payout Ratio	Total dividends paid/Net income	Green	Return on Capital Employed	Earnings before interest and taxes/(Total assets - Current liabilities)	Green
Earnings per Share Ratio	Net income after tax - Preferred stock dividends/Average number of common shares outstanding	Green	Return on Net Assets (RONA)	Net profit/(Fixed assets + Net working capital)	Green
Fixed Asset Turnover Ratio	Net annual sales/(Gross fixed asset - Accumulated depreciation)	Green	Gross Profit Ratio	(Sales – (Direct materials + Direct Labor + Overhead))/Sales	Green

FIGURE 2.16   Financial ratios.

- **Performance ratio.** This is used to measure a company's performance through various analyses including Return on Capital Employed (ROCE), Return on Sales (ROS), and Return on Investment (ROI) [22].
- **Efficiency ratio.** This ratio is used to determine how effectively the company has used its assets—land, machinery, etc—and its people. Sales Per Employee (SPE), Profit Per Employee (PPE) and Sales Per Square Meter (SPM).
- **Current ratio.** This is the relative proportion of an entity's current assets to its current liabilities, and is intended to show the ability of an entity to pay for its current liabilities with its current assets. This is also known as working capital ratio. A working capital ratio of less than 1.0 is a strong indicator that there will be liquidity problems, while a ratio in the vicinity of 2.0 is considered to represent good short-term liquidity.
- **Financial structure ratio.** Financial structure refers to the way in which the company finances itself. Gearing or debt to equity ratio is one such example.
- **Investors' ratio.** This indicates the return on the investment made by the shareholders in the company. Earnings Per Share (EPS) or P/E ratio is a good example.

Inter-company benchmarking is a variation on cross-sectional analysis. This involves an analysis of similar companies, typically in the same industry segment, but this can be extended to compare with other industries as well. A good benchmarking of one company's business can open up several improvement opportunities or merger and acquisition decisions.

HUMAN RESOURCES

People make the dream of a company happen. I was intrigued to learn from Mr. N.R. Narayana Murthy, the co-founder and mentor of Infosys, how he practiced his people vision: "My biggest asset is all my employees who walk out of the gate every evening and I wait for them to come back to me the next morning" [23]. The team who is responsible for finding, developing and making the best use of them is the Human Resources Management team. The purpose of the Human Resources (HR) function is to enhance the people individually and as a team member for the success of the company. The HR department activities cover the following areas:

Employee hiring. This is one of the major activities of the HR function. They are responsible for HR planning and recruitment to fill up vacancies, and they create job specifications, induct new employees, create and implement a people development framework, take decisions on employee relocation and termination, etc.

Performance management. HR creates a performance management framework and a performance management policy, oversees the performance process, ensures fairness in execution, and creates a training plan for people development.

Employee development. People development is the prime responsibility of Human Resources. Employee skills are defined as per the career development framework and HR identifies and ensures employees are trained as per the skill development framework.

Employee reward and recognition. HR ensures employees are motivated for a long-term relationship with the company. The cost of attrition of employees is very high as it takes significant time and money to source, interview, hire and train an employee. A new employee may also need some time to become fully productive. All of these are a significant cost for the employer. So, HR ensures they have the right mechanism to recognize good work and appropriate awards or rewards are given to deserving employees.

Employee relations. HR manages formal and informal relations with individuals or trade unions, administers equal opportunities and creates the right communication mechanism internally and externally.

Health, safety and welfare. HR ensures the right work environment for the employees. This includes health and safety programs, welfare schemes and grievance systems.

The key aims of HR are to create an employee-friendly work environment, create better work opportunities and design programs to keep employees motivated. Though the compensation structure has been created since the abolition of slavery, not many companies have successfully designed overall monetary and non-monetary benefits. Fair compensation may compensate for employees, labor but it doesn't necessarily compensate the company. Employees are part of the company's overall success, which justifies their rewards as the company grows.

Most organizations use an HR portal which provides the single source of all the HR services. The next generation of HR initiatives will come from the effective use of technology. HR will learn from social network sites with the maturity of data privacy and security. Though this looks far sighted and many countries are already opposed to HR making decisions based on social network data, I strongly believe it is just a matter of time before this becomes the most effective tool for HR decisions.

Another area which will increasingly make use of technology in HR is compliance. More and more regulatory compliance needs corporate data transparency, effective management of data, data analysis for more business insights and reporting to the regulatory authorities in a timely manner. The regulatory changes will ask companies to make the information available for frequent submissions.

Chapter 3

Technology Basics—An Introduction

PACKAGED AND CUSTOM DEVELOPED TECHNOLOGY SOLUTIONS

David is a senior director responsible for managing field force realignment. At the end of the quarter, he wants to analyze Rx data (prescription data) and market trends for several products, and also to tweak campaigns based on data-based analysis. When David asks his Information Technology (IT) team to make this happen, he finds out that it takes several weeks, if not months, to get the data put onto the IT systems for David and his team to look at. After doing all the hard work to build a strategy that needs to be implemented within days to have an impact on the market, he cannot believe that the IT department will become a bottleneck. When he tries further reasoning, David gets completely lost in the IT jargon—databases, DW, ETL, BI, data cleansing, fields, columns, down-stream systems, SDLC, interfaces, and so on!

Christina has an idea for an IT system that would help consolidate KOL (Key Opinion Leader) management activities for cross-branding, idea sharing, executing surveys and creating a single interface between her company and KOLs, and would eliminate the chaos of multiple company representatives working independently with the KOL. Christina works on a charter and calls her IT colleague, Sunder, to initiate this IT project. She hasn't worked on any IT system development projects on her own and wants to give it a go. She realizes after a few days that it might have been a foolhardy move! The IT team does not seem to understand anything she is trying to explain and asks questions that are either too obvious about very basic business needs or they ask totally irrelevant questions. Christina keeps calm; she tries to educate the IT team members. She is happy when the team finally compiles all her requirements in a document they call URS (User Requirement Specification), a nice

Pharma's Prescription. http://dx.doi.org/10.1016/B978-0-12-407662-4.00003-9

meaningful name. But the joy is very shortlived—Sunder asks her to review a huge document after several weeks of finalizing the URS.

"What's this, Sunder?" asks Christina.

Sunder explains that this 200-page document is an FRS (Functional Requirement Specification). He asks Christina to review this in as much detail as possible because she won't be able to modify anything after this point, when IT coding would be implemented into the document. Politely Sunder tells her that he typically reviews the FRS himself for the areas he has business knowledge of, but as KOL is something very new to him, he wants Christina to review and approve it instead.

Christina is lost. She is overwhelmed with her day job. The IT development job has now turned out to be very complicated; on top of that, Sunder tells her that the IT contractors cannot work on the job until the FRS sign-off but will have to be paid in the meantime. Christina now deeply regrets embarking on the KOL management system project!

Does this sound familiar? This is the story of almost all business teams who are working with IT teams on a day to day basis. This chapter intends to help articulate some of the basics of IT which will make business stakeholders like Christina get conversant with the IT processes, expectations from business, timeline, various options, etc. and which will help prepare them when discussing projects with IT teams so that they are not caught off-guard.

IT has been around for many years. IT has been excellent for process automation to improve productivity, speed up tasks, increase accuracy of outputs, and it provides the possibility for structuring information for easy access and creating business insights; it deploys algorithms to build an insight out of plain data; and it gives intelligence-based computation to learn and solve business problems that are otherwise difficult to execute manually. Decades ago, IT systems were delivered only through large computer systems using punch cards. IT has continually evolved at an ever-growing pace to use more intuitive programming languages and easy to use interfaces. The evolution of IT in the last 15 years has developed from the use of punch cards to machine level languages, fourth generation languages, object orientated programming, WYSIWYG (what you see is what you get), mobile computing, artificial intelligence, SaaS products and many more (see Figure 3.1).

There are many complexities involved at every level of IT but a business partner developing an IT system doesn't need to know all of that. They only need to know answers to some basic questions such as:

- What is IT, when do I need IT and what can IT do for me?
- What do IT teams do to build and manage systems?

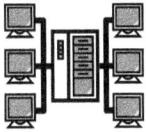

Mainframe Systems	**Personal Computers**	**Open Systems**	**Cloud-Based Systems**
Large, high capacity, powerful computing machines; Procedural programming capability; Character-based user interface through dumb terminals	Small, portable machines with significant computing power; Object oriented programming capability; Rich Graphical User Interface (GUI)	Scalable, high capacity, high performance machines; Advanced messaging and communication protocols; Flexible architecture	Flexible and on demand computing power; Ready to use business applications; System integration capability to other system components

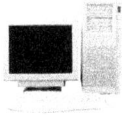

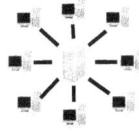

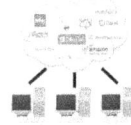

FIGURE 3.1   Technology evolution.

- What do IT systems look like and what are the different types of IT systems?
- How do I ensure the IT solution being developed will work for me?
- What support does IT need from the business team?

Let us try to find these answers.

What is IT, When Do I Need IT and What Can IT Do for Me?

In simple terms, IT is often used to automate repeatable business processes and execute them faster and error-free. If you create a large amount of paper-based content that needs to refer back to the paper work in the future (e.g. batch manufacturing records, lab notebooks), IT can help make them paperless. IT algorithms can solve complex math problems in no time. IT programs, once built, can predict business situations through complex analysis of data. If you need to exchange information and collaborate with other group members or partners within the company or outside, or if you want to harness the power of the world-wide-web, IT can help.

What Do IT Teams Do to Build and Manage Systems?

IT teams develop applications, make them useful to the users, support the system, resolve user's issues and modify applications as needed by the users. This whole life cycle is known as system development, support and maintenance. This IT application cannot work on its own and needs other systems to support it. The overall system has several components—infrastructure, operating system, platform and business application.

Computer infrastructure (server hardware, desktops, laptops, computer networks, routers), operating systems (Windows or Unix), technology platforms (Oracle databases, SAP installations, application servers, web servers, mobile device management systems, email systems) and business applications are built using all the above components to execute a business process, e.g. travel and expense. The user only sees the business application which is typically installed on the user's device or accessed through their devices.

This is just like building a kitchen to cook a meal. If we start from the beginning, we first need to create a house foundation (infrastructure), a kitchen (operating system), and we need a combination of utensils, water, electricity, etc. (the business application). The output is the meal enjoyed by the user—similar to the travel and expenses report created by the IT application. The kitchen cannot stand without a proper foundation or infrastructure and the meal cannot be cooked without the help of utensils or applications. The house structure needs to be maintained by applying various chemicals and modified as and when the dwellers want. Similarly, IT systems and applications need to be taken care of throughout their entire life cycle, which is known as application support and maintenance. To build and maintain a house, we all need to follow some standards and abide by township and other regulations. Similarly, IT system development follows standard processes and several regulations imposed by the health authorities, e.g. Computer System Validation (CSV), 21 CFR Part 11 for electronic signature and electronic records, etc. IT systems are frequently audited by the authorities to check that they are functioning correctly just like townships regularly inspect houses.

Let's look at IT system development, support and maintenance work in more depth. The most commonly used software development processes are "Waterfall Method" and "Agile Method".

Waterfall Method

This method comprises various phases—plan (idea or charter), requirements, design, build, test, roll-out, and support (see Figure 3.2). If the system supports regulated business processes, it needs to follow computer system validation guidelines as well. The basic idea here is to complete one set of activities that drive the next step. The output of one step becomes the input to the next. It's one-directional, as in the way water falls. For example, the requirement needs to be completed and finalized before the system can be designed; the design needs to be completed before the system development, and so on. This is the traditional model

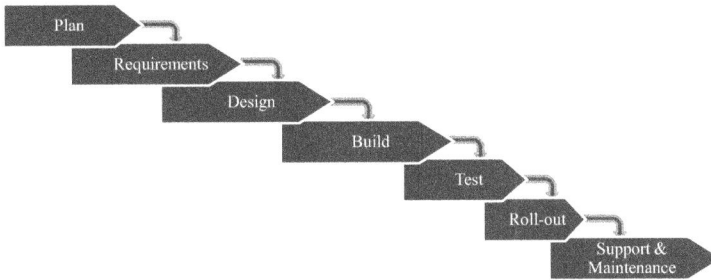

FIGURE 3.2 Waterfall method of software development.

adopted for most system development—hardware and software—and is still the most commonly used model. This is most suitable when we know exactly what we want or when the level of ambiguity is relatively low.

Plan. The IT system development starts with a high-level idea definition and a plan to execute it. This consists of crystalizing an idea, which could be to identify a business problem or bring in a new capability. This idea gets discussed with various potential users and IT teams to develop a project charter. If the system is large enough, it should go through a business case development exercise to identify business value and compute Return on Investment (ROI). Once the plan is approved, the next phase, requirement gathering, is executed.

Requirements. The IT team organizes meetings, conferences and workshops with the business users to understand the objectives, needs, expectations, and review prior documentation, create business scenarios, prototypes, etc. so as to understand the IT application functionalities. These requirements are documented, reviewed and approved as the User Requirement Specification (URS) or Business Requirement Specification (BRS). The IT team takes the URS as their foundation document and details out functionalities exactly the way the system will behave in a Functional Requirements Specification (FRS) document. While the URS is more aligned to what the business user would like to see in the system, the FRS is more aligned to the needs from a systems perspective. The FRS is the input to the technology teams to create the system architecture and various integration components, and to design a system which can be built by the coders. These documents are to get clarity on the requirements, get consensus from all the parties involved and help avoid any future misunderstanding between teams. The best practice is to create a traceability matrix which traces each business requirement across several artifacts developed in the various Software Development Life Cycle (SDLC) phases. Once the requirements have been defined and documented, the documents are signed off and a baseline is created for future reference and to track changes, if any. The URS and FRS definition is the most critical step in the entire SDLC process. Any error in the requirement definition is spread through all other phases and reflects in the end product as well. Also, any error at this stage is the most difficult and costly to detect and fix at later stages. While the IT industry has many processes and techniques to manage this effectively, the industry statistics do not show very convincing data—only little over 55% of requirements are delivered in the final product. So, all stakeholders involved at this stage should increase their focus on the subsequent development phases as well to ensure the right delivery of the end product.

Design. In the design phase, FRS is used to design various parts of the system—Architecture, Proof of Concepts (PoC), Database Objects, User Interfaces, Connections, and Application Program, etc. Generally, Technical Architects, Database Modelers, and Technical Analysts are involved in design activities. The outcome of this phase is the design document which serves as the instruction to the software developers and helps them configure, code, and test the system. During this phase, the IT team may need further verification or clarification on requirements.

Build. Once the design document(s) are available, the developers are involved in coding the various parts of the system. This phase is known as build. It is useful to organize intermittent demonstration of the parts of the system to the users for their early feedback, especially the user interface design. This early engagement can ease the deployment of the system to the users as they have already seen some parts and given their concurrences. The build phase is the most effort-intensive phase in the SDLC process, consumes most IT bandwidth and is also the longest of all SDLC phases. Once the coding is complete, each developer performs unit testing—to test the individual components of the software. The combination of coding and unit testing is referred to as "build". At the end of this phase, the unit tested code is ready for the subsequent phase, called test.

Test. This phase comprises several tests including the integration test (IT), system test (ST), and user acceptance test (UAT). The integration test is to ensure that various components can work together. The system test confirms that the integrated system meets all the functional requirements defined in the FRS. The UAT conforms to the

URS and is usually done by the actual users of the system. Test scripts are created for each requirement and tested using test data. To ensure ruggedness of the system, boundary conditions, complex conditions and hypothetical conditions, there are several other non-functional tests. Further tests such as the performance test, stress or load test, and security test are conducted. The outcome of this phase is a completely tested system that is ready for business users. UAT is done as the last step in the process and once this is out of the way, the business users certify the system ready to move into the production environment for the entire business community to use. The production environment of the system is the final technology environment to host the application for the end users, but there are other environments to create for development work and tests. Development is done using a development environment, and tests are done using a test environment. These environments are created as per the technology capacity requirements and match the user's profile—developers for the development team, testers for the testing environment and business users for the production environment.

Roll-out. During this phase, the system is installed on the production environment. Once installed, a round of sanity tests, also known as smoke tests, is performed to check if the system performs as required and is operating as intended. Once the verification process is over, the system is handed over to the business users for normal business operations. Generally, roll-out is followed by post-deployment warranty support for a defined period. During this period, members of the IT team stand by for any clarifications or corrections required.

Support. This is the ongoing phase after the system goes live in the production environment. During this phase, the IT team provides Level 1, Level 2 and Level 3 system supports to the system users. Level 1 support includes receiving and resolving a simple user query without spending much time. This can be done through a phone conversation or sending pre-scripted resolutions to the users. But if the user query issues cannot be solved quickly and need more investigation to find a resolution, it gets categorized as Level 2. This support team solves the issues that can be solved without changing the system. The Level 3 support handles issues or requests that can only be resolved through changing the system. Changes to the system mean the IT team has to go through the entire software development life cycle process—gather or clarify requirements, update the design document, make changes to the code, test it (both for the changes made as well as related functionalities that would have had an impact because of this change). Level 3 support is also classified as "system maintenance" as it involves making changes to the system.

The IT system keeps a lean team for continuous support and maintenance work. This team gets augmented to carry out system enhancement activities. It's always likely to get several user requests to modify or add functionalities as they use the system again and again. These requests are handled as "system enhancement" and get executed under the system enhancement budget.

Several forms of input need to be considered to make the enhancements available to the users. Releases to the production environments are prescheduled as the release demands a production system shut-down during which users can't use the system.

Agile Method

The Agile Method is another model that is prevalent in the industry. It is in many ways different from the Waterfall Method and follows the application development in relay sprints with smaller parts getting built and delivered to get early user feedback. The basic principle in this very modern idea is to provide freedom to the users to ask for more and more functionalities as they start seeing some output. It is hard to visualize unknowns completely as in the case of the development of the Waterfall Method. The Agile Method, as the name suggests, provides far more flexibility in finalizing the end product. Hence, the model propagates building in small iterations and adds more functions as users see things in the iterations. This is extremely suitable for the development of new solutions using newer technologies which have not yet been fully tested and therefore have uncertain final outcomes. I personally think this is the model to go with, given that technology moves so fast and locking-in requirements several months ahead of time doesn't give the highest level of user satisfaction. Most of the individual steps are similar to the steps defined above and hence the diagram in Figure 3.3 is self-explanatory.

There is of course much more to these processes—this is just an overview and a highly simplified view of how the systems are developed and maintained. However, this level of detail provides sufficient knowledge to IT newbies.

Now that we know how the systems are developed and maintained, it may be worthwhile to explore what's inside these systems.

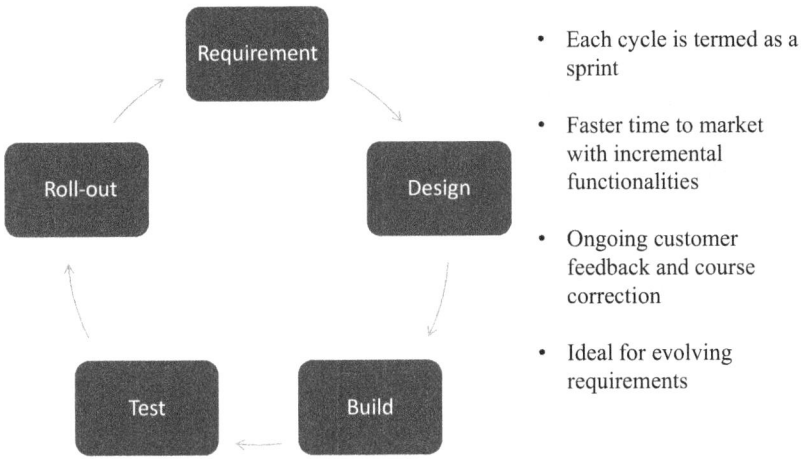

- Each cycle is termed as a sprint

- Faster time to market with incremental functionalities

- Ongoing customer feedback and course correction

- Ideal for evolving requirements

FIGURE 3.3   Agile method of software development.

What Do IT Systems Look Like and What are the Different Types of IT Systems?

IT systems generally comprise hardware, an operating system and software. All of these components have evolved significantly over a period of time to bring in greater capacity, flexibility, performance and reliability. The IT department manages all of these. They need to procure and configure the hardware, buy licenses for use, install operating systems and middleware components and develop and maintain business applications, using this infrastructure. Again, all of these topics are big enough to have separate chapters. To keep it simple, however, I will only explain the aspects with regard to the business application and will briefly discuss what goes into such software. At a very high level, the entire system has three basic layers—Presentation Layer, Business Layer and Data Layer. Through the evolution process, these layers have been broken up further to take advantage of the evolving technologies and to meet specific business needs (see Figure 3.4).

Presentation Layer. This is also known as the UI (User Interface). This layer accepts information from users, relays the information to the next layer (Business Layer), and returns the results to the user. This layer has a direct impact on usability, productivity and adoption of a system by the user. The UI is a critical aspect in the success or failure of an application and most projects engage specialists with user

Business Application System

REQUEST ────────────────→

| Presentation Layer | Business Layer | Data Layer |

Enter Data

Receive Results

Business user

←──────── RESPONSE ────────

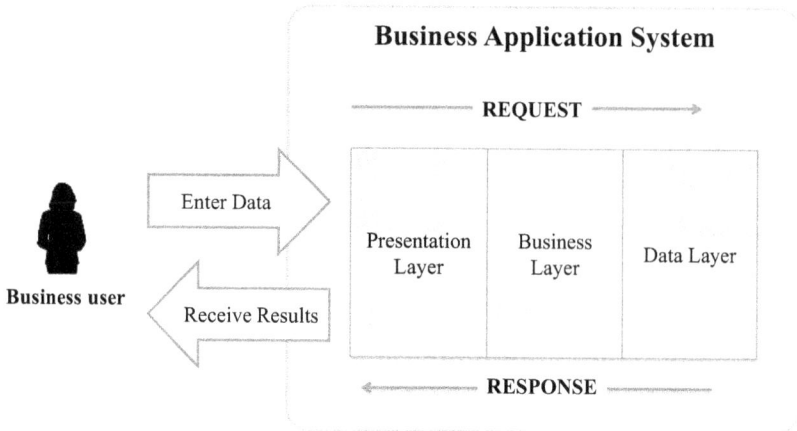

FIGURE 3.4 Business application.

experience (UX)—experts like UX designer and UX architect—to ensure UI is intuitive and suits the needs of the user group.

Business Layer. This is the heart of the system and it stores the functional logic of the business application. Legacy systems generally use procedural language which flows from top to bottom to execute a set of instructions. Modern systems use object oriented languages that build logically independent components called objects and invoke these components as required. The Business Layer exchanges information with the Presentation Layer to interact with the end users and exchanges information with the Data Layer to store or retrieve data.

Data Layer. This layer comprises data stores (commonly known as databases) and functions that help store or retrieve data on these data stores. Data stores have evolved substantially over time. The primitive data stores were simple text files that were indexed to help speed up the data operations (Insert/Modify/Delete/Retrieve). Data for separate functions was stored on separate files. Special files were used to establish relationships between different files. Modern systems started storing data on tables and managed the relationships between tables. These became easier to work with and faster to operate. Generally, these were referred to as RDBMS (Relational Database Management System). Further evolution allowed systems to organize and store data using object models. Designing an optimal database is critical to the performance and maintainability of a system in the long run.

Over time, technology has evolved and led to the development of different types of systems, each with their own benefits. The following section describes several system types.

Mainframe/Legacy Systems. These are the oldest IT systems that were the first widely used systems for running businesses. In these systems, the entire software resides and runs on the mainframe machines. These machines are hooked up to terminals (also called dumb terminals) only to display information and accept inputs from the user. Generally, these systems had a language to design the screens, e.g. CICS, and code to write the business logic, e.g. COBOL and PL1. The databases to store the information were DB2 or SUPRA. The mainframe systems have mostly been replaced by the modern systems.

Desktop Application. These systems took advantage of the computing power of a personal computer and hence the ability to work without having to log on to the mainframes. It enabled rich graphical user interfaces and provided much of the flexibility that was previously missing. These systems worked well in isolation, e.g. independent research or data entry, and with minimal data transfer needs. However, over time these systems ended up with several constraints related to software distribution, the inability to share and the choking of network bandwidth due to sharing of large files across users. Most of these systems were developed in BASIC, C, POWER BUILDER, VISUAL BASIC with local databases such as SYBASE, ACCESS, and MY SQL.

Client Server System. With increased internet bandwidth availability and advancement in technologies that could connect software components remotely, most of the desktop systems were replaced with client server systems. The initial variant of the client server system had two parts and was also known as the 2-tier architecture (see Figure 3.5). This architecture required transfer of data to be displayed on the screen as opposed to transferring the entire data store as in the case of sharing data on desktop systems. This allowed several advantages including larger capacity and computing power of a server,

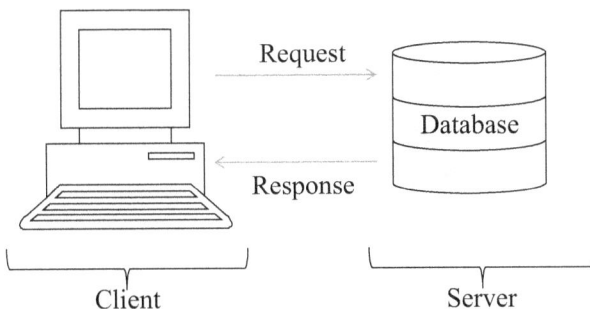

FIGURE 3.5   2-Tier Client Server System Architecture.

ability to share the same data store across several users, and freeing up network bandwidth. However, there were several other problems related to performance—multiple and sustained connections to the server and heavy reliance on database—and software distribution to ensure the compatible version of the software was installed for the client especially for systems with a larger user base.

To solve some of the problems inherent to the 2-tier architecture, an additional layer was introduced and a 3-tier architecture was developed (see Figure 3.6). The purpose of the 3-tier architecture was to reduce the number of connections required to the database server, move some of the business logic to the application server, relegate the role of the database to store and retrieve data, and improve the overall performance and maintainability of the system.

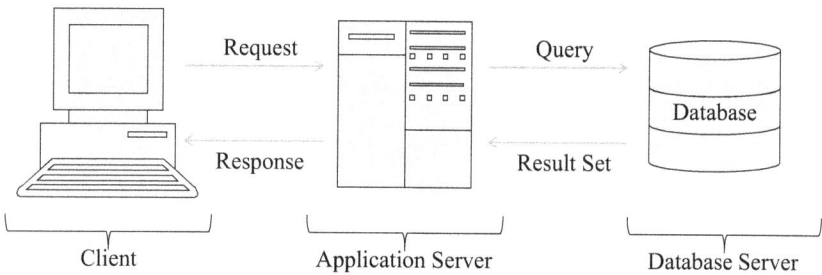

FIGURE 3.6   3-Tier Client Server System Architecture.

Technology evolves very rapidly and a huge number of programming languages were in play including some of the older ones. Most of the messaging systems and communication protocols to manage interactions between various tiers were developed and matured during this time. Client server systems had presentation layers developed using languages such as VISUAL BASIC and POWER BUILDER or later using HTML, CSS, and XML that could reduce the footprint of the components to be installed on the desktop. A host of scripting languages also came into place to add additional functions and features on the screens. Business layers were mostly developed in Java and .NET. and the Data Layer comprised various types of databases including SQL Server, SYBASE and ORACLE.

Web-Based System. The advantages of having the software installed and run on a server and the widespread availability of the internet led

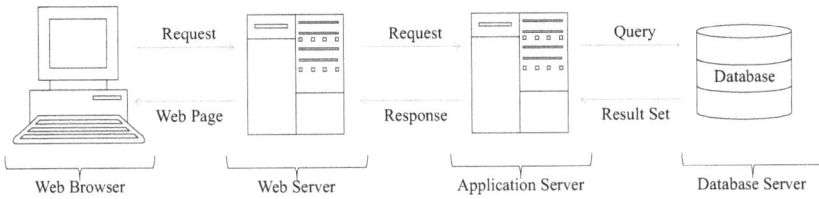

FIGURE 3.7   n-Tier Client Server System Architecture.

the way to moving the entire presentation layer onto the servers. These systems do not have any software installed on the desktops—they usually only have a link or a URL (something like http:\\xxx.yyy.zzz) that points to the Web Server. Since this introduces another tier and the number of tiers could potentially increase depending on the capacity, performance and load balancing needs, this architecture was also called the n-tier architecture (see Figure 3.7).

Web Servers serve web pages that act as the Presentation Layer and are connected to the Application Servers that act as the Business Layer that in turn are connected to the Databases. Most modern systems are web-based systems. The biggest advantage of these systems is the ability to manage the software. Since there is no software to be installed on the desktop, problems related to software distribution were almost completely resolved. This is when the internet also boomed to develop millions of websites—some of them static (only serving to provide information to the users) while others were dynamic with the ability to work as an application.

Cloud-Based System. Consider a business application like Customer Resource Management (CRM) system for company A and another one for company B. Typically, these systems would be developed according to the specific needs of company A and company B. And these systems would also be installed in data centers owned by the individual companies. The separate infrastructure leads to very high technology cost. One option to reduce cost is to share infrastructure. So, what if company A and company B both want to share the infrastructure of CRM software? Furthermore, what if we allow more such companies to share the same software installation? With technological advancements this is possible without creating interference of business between each other, and no mixing of their data or information at all. This allows individual companies to get rid of their individual data centers and hence reduce major costs. The key concepts of a Cloud-Based System are multi-tenancy (multiple companies rent the same IT system) and rapid deployment as they are generally out of the box (OOTB); functionalities are readily available and do not need to be developed for every company. This reduces the hardware footprint.

Today, while the technology is evolving, several companies are embracing Cloud-Based systems.

So, yes, in more than one way, there is a lot involved in building a system which works for the business. While IT teams decide on the technology design, the business team needs to help them with functionalities, data, performance needs, security and compliance matters. With this high-level technology understanding, I'm sure business stakeholders will now appreciate the questions that IT teams ask that sound very silly otherwise.

How do I Ensure the IT Solution being Developed will Work for Me?

It depends entirely on how well IT and business work together for it to be a success. Technology-driven solutions should not be the responsibility of IT or business alone—both need to do it together. The industry has matured in processes, tools, templates and accelerators to make the project successful every time, but industry data does not support it. A recent study showed that over 66% of software projects' costs overrun, 33% of projects had schedule overrun and 17% fall short of values [24].

IT solution development is a combination of art and science—mathematics and imagination are both equally important. There are many reasons why a combination of art and science does not work in a project situation—I will give the top three.

Firstly, ensure the requirements are good. If there is just one thing that I would recommend, it would be to help the IT team define the requirements—work out the details, provide illustrations, clarify doubts and go through prototyping. If the outcome of the requirements document can be used to test the end product completely or map the functions of an existing software product, you have achieved a large part of your goal.

Secondly, ensure you maintain a constant touch point with the IT team throughout the entire SDLC phase. There is no need to micromanage the IT team, but it is important to get involved in the governance process. Over half of IT projects go through project management challenges that make the schedule and cost overrun. Business and IT leaders should form joint governance teams and jointly own the right delivery schedule. I also recommend having a business quality control person spend enough bandwidth to review deliverables and milestones to catch any problem upfront.

Thirdly, the communication between all the relevant stakeholders needs to be very well established. Many projects fail because the stakeholders are set the wrong expectations, which creates serious issues when the system is delivered. One such example is that the business team and IT team must communicate and jointly pick the right technology solution to avoid confusion and rework later in the project.

What Support Does IT Need from the Business Team?

No IT project can be successful without business support and participation. In saying this, I'm referring to IT-driven business solutions, not just any IT project. The IT team needs support from the business users throughout the entire SDLC phases. However, the involvement levels vary significantly between the phases. For example, requirement gathering and UAT phases need the most involvement—design and build need the least. The exact effort depends on the size and complexity of the project, but the table below provides a ball-park estimate of the business team effort spread across the SDLC phases.

Requirements	Design	Build	Test	Rollout
60	10	5	20	5

Business user involvement greatly depends on the type of the IT project; however, at a high level, the key activities include the following:

- Requirements phase: Interviews, workshops, proto-typing, existing systems and processes demonstration, document reviews and sign-off
- Design: Requirement clarification, test case development and review, user interface (screen views or prototype) review, document reviews and sign-off
- Build: Document reviews and sign-off
- Test: Review test results, perform user acceptance tests, product sign-off
- Deploy: Sanity tests—conduct a sample test of the system functionalities as users would use them to certify the system works in the production environment.

While the basic elements of the software development remain the same, different methodologies require a varied level of effort from the business users. For example, the Agile Method involves small sprints and demands a higher level of involvement from the business users to validate requirements, prototypes, and test and end results in each sprint. Similarly, most of the cloud-based systems adopt OOTB and the custom code strategy. While OOTB can be configured very quickly, custom coding may require a number of iterations before the design can be finalized.

The process rigor changes for the regulated and business critical applications. These applications follow Computer System Validation (CSV) process. The next section describes this process in more detail.

COMPUTER SYSTEM VALIDATION

Computer System Validation (CSV) is the process of establishing documented evidence, which provides a high degree of assurance that a specific process will consistently deliver a computer system as its predetermined specifications and quality attributes [25].

The necessity of performing validation of IT systems, personnel training and maintaining proper documentation is a normal business strategy today and not just a regulatory requirement. The cost of non-compliance is huge and it is always beneficial to follow CSV on a day to day basis.

The pharmaceutical IT is different from the regular IT because of the regulatory complexities. This increases documentation, reviews and approval processes and increases both time and cost. However, this process rigor helps getting the product right the first time which in turn ensures faster speed to market and reduction in re-work cost. The CSV follows a 4-tier functional architecture which is in line with the USFDA guidelines (see Figure 3.8). These layers are: (1) Compliance policy understanding and application, (2) Process documentation—development, package implementation, maintenance, etc., (3) Process aids—SOP, checklist, guideline and deliverables, and (4) Maintenance of project records.

The validation process ensures the right solution is built and delivered to the users. This process answers several critical questions around five areas—planning, risk management, qualification, documentation and traceability.

Validation planning:
- What are the critical business and quality aspects of the system?
- What will be the validation approach and scope of validation activities?

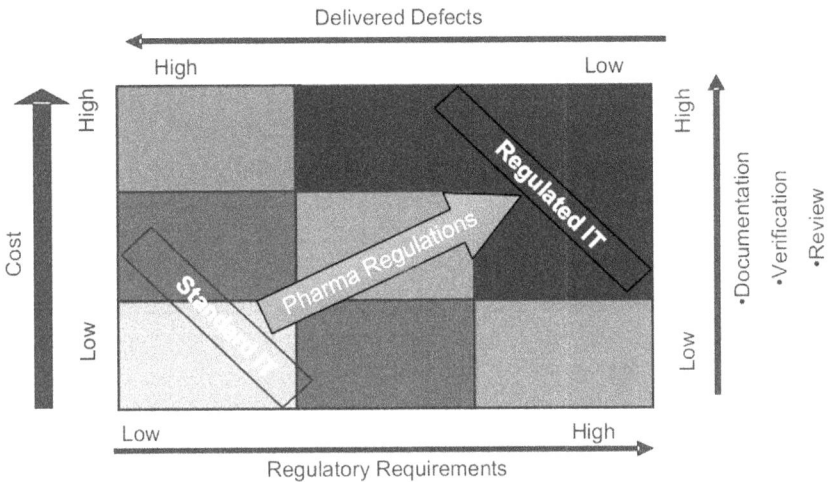

FIGURE 3.8 Regulated IT.

- What will be the validation deliverables, who will be responsible for them, and what will be the acceptance criteria for the validated system?
- What processes will be followed to ensure high quality?

System risk assessment:

- Are the user requirements captured accurately?
- Are the URS (User Requirement Specification) and FS (Functional Specification) documents complete with all details?
- What will be the PQ (Performance Qualfication) test environment and what will be the critical test cases?
- Are functional requirements mapping to URS?
- What will be the IQ (Installation Qualification) and OQ (Operational Qualification) test environment and critical test cases?
- Do the detailed design specifications cover all the functionalities?

System qualification:

- How will the IQ, OQ and PQ plans be evaluated and approved?
- Are DQ (Design Qualification) components installed properly?
- Are the IQ, OQ and PQ protocols complete and reviewed?
- Do the IQ and OQ results establish with documented evidence that the design and functionality of the system are as desired?
- Has the UAT environment been set up adequately to mimic the actual production environment?

Documentation:
- Has the validation plan been prepared, reviewed and agreed by all stakeholders?
- Is the validation report updated at each stage?
- Is the validation documentation complete?

Traceability:
- Can the detailed design be traced to the functional and user specifications?
- Can the test cases for IQ be mapped to the detailed design?
- Can the test cases for OQ be traced to the functional specification (FS)?
- Can the test cases for PQ be mapped to the User Requirement Specifications (URS)?

The CSV process starts with the validation master plan which addresses validation-specific activities to be performed at each of the validation life cycle stages, identifies roles and responsibilities and defines validation deliverables. The compliance process consists of four main stages and several sub-categories.

1. Validation Strategy
2. Validation execution and verification: user requirements, functional requirements, design, IQ/OQ/PQ
3. Validation summary report and recommendation for release
4. Validation evaluation and recommendation for ongoing activities.

Validation Strategy

This is the first stage of the validation process. This can be broken into two phases for a large program or all-encompassing single phase. The purpose of the phase is to create a master validation strategy or a master validation plan for the entire program which might have several projects under the same program. This is a strategy or master plan as it may consist of several sub-plans. If there is a multi-country ERP roll-out over a couple of years, the master plan describes the validation strategy for all the countries and a validation plan gets created to execute validation activities in each country. So the master plan is the overall validation strategy with several validation plans within. This is the approach I have taken when consulting with several large pharmaceutical companies but a company may have a specific approach in their quality management system which needs to be followed. This company-specific alignment of the process is one of the key activities in this stage.

I recommend using the V-Model of validation for CSV compliance (see Figure 3.9). This is aligned with the FDA CSV guidelines and ensures validation work throughout the entire SDLC (Software Development Life Cycle) process stages.

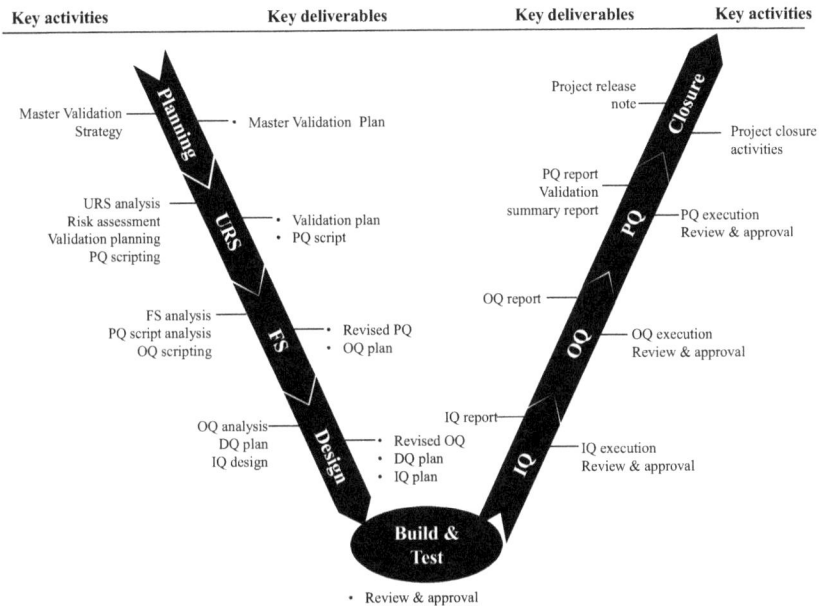

| Key activities | Key deliverables | Key deliverables | Key activities |

Master Validation Strategy

Planning

- Master Validation Plan

Project release note

Closure

Project closure activities

URS analysis
Risk assessment
Validation planning
PQ scripting

URS

- Validation plan
- PQ script

PQ report
Validation summary report

PQ

PQ execution
Review & approval

FS analysis
PQ script analysis
OQ scripting

FS

- Revised PQ
- OQ plan

OQ report

OQ

OQ execution
Review & approval

OQ analysis
DQ plan
IQ design

Design

- Revised OQ
- DQ plan
- IQ plan

IQ report

IQ

IQ execution
Review & approval

Build & Test

- Review & approval

FIGURE 3.9   V-Model of validation.

The **validation plan** helps define the rationale of the validation approach and the scope of validation activities for a project as it:

- Defines validation activities at each stage of validation which is aligned with the software development life cycle stages
- Defines in detail the acceptance criteria of the deliverables and the system
- Defines roles and responsibilities for all the activities. This should include the executers, reviewers, approvers and the change controller
- Defines documentation procedure
- Defines deliverables at various life cycle stages including the validation summary report.

The validation plan should describe details about the new software development validation or, major enhancement validation or small changes in validation processes, as applicable, as the complexities and number of deliverables vary significantly. The validation of a new software development is a very involved process, whereas the enhancement mostly needs several modifications of the existing documents. So, the plan should give details of the differences which will reduce the execution ambiguity. A validation plan document needs to be created and signed off at this stage.

Validation Execution and Verification

The validation execution and verification stage starts with the user requirements and ends with the performance qualification execution, and reports the results.

The user requirements analysis includes a review and approval of the URS document, identifies critical business needs and creates Performance Qualification (PQ) test plans or scripts to ensure those requirements are tested and delivered. This also includes reviewing the requirement traceability document.

The system risk assessment and aligning quality goals is a critical element not only for the quality and compliance perspective but also for ensuring the delivery of the right business solution. This is a highly debatable area and I have heard many arguments on whether the quality team should be part of the IT solution development discussions and decisions. One such debate was at a top 10 pharmaceutical company who was rolling out a global customer relationship management (CRM) solution to the field force. The quality team was short of bandwidth, like always, and they decided to advise from outside without getting involved at the beginning of the project. The solution team happily agreed to this as they never thought the quality and compliance team was a value added service to the project team. The outcome was disastrous. This large project had over USD 100 million investment and close to two years of project work. But when the time came for the validation summary report by their quality and compliance team, they were shocked to see the level of misalignment with their internal policies and procedures, including the lack of validation deliverables. The solution could not be put into operation. They had to bring in an independent validation team, an army of people in fact, to fix this problem. The project overran by nine months with a 40% in project cost. The business opportunity loss was not quantified, but all agreed that it was a huge amount. The competitive edge they wanted to create through this automation was completely lost. This is one experience I always share with the project stakeholders when they question quality and compliance team involvement in solution planning. My advice is to involve them as early as the project definition phase.

The **FS** phase is an important phase from the validation perspective to ensure all the requirements are translated into application functionalities. As the industry data shows, many business requirements get dropped in this phase due to a lack of understanding of the requirements. A validation team reviews the FS document, traceability of functional specification to the URS and gives the go-ahead to move into the detailed design phase. It's also good to review the PQ test plan or scripts created in the URS phase and update them based on the functional specification details. The deliverables include revised PQ plan or scripts, the operation qualification (OQ) plan or scripts and the FS analysis report. Validation leaders with a good understanding of technology can create wonders in this phase.

The design, build, and test phases are very technical. The validation team involvements are greatly reduced. However, the validation team ensures standards are followed, the right documents are created and adherence to functional specifications and design traceability are maintained.

The following activities are executed in this phase:

- Review of system design/configuration specifications and associated documentation. Ensure they are in line with documentation standards
- Review traceability of URS to FS and designs; ensure closure of any gaps
- Review and approve test plan/scripts. Ensure test plan covers all design/functional requirements
- Perform risk analysis of system test scripts if risk-based test method is used in the project
- Ensure coding standard is used, code verification is performed and unit tests are done
- Verify system test results; verify integration test results.

Update the validation summary report with the activities and results completed.

Once the project team completes the system development activities including system and integration tests, the validation team may take over over the independent IQ, OQ and PQ execution. An independent execution is advised for the larger, complex and highly regulated systems and it can be optimized greatly for other projects. The optimization is through executing some of the validation activities by the project teams and the independent validation manager reviews and approves the output. This saves time and money while all the validation tasks are executed.

The **Installation Qualification (IQ)** phase ensures all the system components are installed as defined in the design document. This is a checklist-driven exercise to ensure components are installed and tested and functionalities are established. The IQ result document is created; once approved, the system is installed in the staging environment to carry out OQ and PQ. The staging environment is an environment which mimics the production environment but is a scaled-down version.

Installation protocol is finalized at this stage and approved by the validation team. The IQ test result document is created and the validation summary report is updated with the IQ details.

The **Operation Qualification (OQ)** ensures the system performs as per the functional specifications. All the functionalities defined in the FS should be tested to establish the OQ.

To establish the OQ, the system needs to be connected to all interfaces. The actual interfaces may be difficult to establish in the staging environment but a simulated environment needs to be created to achieve this:

- Execute OQ test scripts and document OQ results
- Update validation report with OQ results.

The **Performance Qualification (PQ)** ensures the system performs as per the User Requirement Specifications. The following activities are performed at this stage:

- Support users for executing PQ scripts
- Post execution review and approval of PQ protocol
- Prepare the PQ summary report
- Review and approve traceability matrix
- Review and ensure updates to OQ and PQ test plan/scripts if needed
- Ensure completion of pre-release activities
- Update and complete validation summary report.

Validation Summary Report and Recommendation for Release

A formal validation summary report is a must have document for a validated system. This is structured during the validation planning phase, gets updated throughout the entire execution phase, and is finalized in this phase. A product release note which certifies the software product's suitability to get deployed in the production environment is created based on the validation summary report. This report should make very specific "go" or "no-go" recommendation. A "go" recommendation with certain open items with a well-defined closure plan is also acceptable. However, no decision status other than go/no-go is unacceptable.

Validation Evaluation and Recommendation for Ongoing Activities

As a best practice, it is always important to look back and check whether improvements can be made to the validation process and other activities after completing a project. I recommend formalizing this process by introducing a "validation evaluation" phase in the validation process.

Validation of a project is not just a one-off activity. The majority of tasks are done during the validation process but there are continuous activities including change control, training, documentation and modification of validation deliverables as the system goes through changes.

A formal change control board is recommended. This board can control several validated systems. However, a formal process needs to be established and communicated to the project teams to use this service to always maintain the system in the "validated status".

21 CFR PART 11 COMPLIANCE

Information technology automates several processes and helps establish a paperless working environment in several operating areas. A manufacturing shop floor runs with near zero papers with the help of a manufacturing execution system, PLCs; a marketing operation works paperless with digitized content; and test labs run paperless with the help of an Electronic Laboratory Notebook (eLN) and a Laboratory Information Management system (LIMS). With the help of technology the industry has moved towards a paperless work environment, and the health authorities have progressed too. They accept electronic signatures in the submission document instead of a paper-based wet signature using ink. They accept electronic records if they follow the FDA guidelines. The FDA policy on electronic records and electronic signatures is known as 21 CFR Part11.

As per the FDA, the electronic records and electronic signatures are defined below [26]:

- Records that are required to be maintained under predicate rule requirements and that are maintained in electronic format in place of a paper format. On the other hand, records (and any associated signatures) that are not required to be retained under predicate rules, but that are nonetheless maintained in electronic format, are not Part 11 records.

- Records that are required to be maintained under predicate rules, that are maintained in electronic format in addition to paper format, and that are relied on to perform regulated activities.
- Records submitted to the FDA, under predicate rules in electronic format. However, a record that is not itself submitted, but is used in generating a submission, is not a Part 11 record unless it is otherwise required to be maintained under a predicate rule and it is maintained in electronic format.
- Electronic signatures that are intended to be the equivalent of hand-written signatures, initials, and other general signings required by predicate rules. Part 11 signatures include electronic signatures that are used, for example, to document the fact that certain events or actions occurred in accordance with the predicate rule (e.g. approved, reviewed, and verified).

The first action for a pharmaceutical company around Part 11 is to define their own definition of electronic records. I have seen many project teams struggle to find out if their system or part of the system they were developing fell under Part 11 compliance. The simpler rule could be "any record that is subject to regulatory audits or can be used in regulatory submissions, maintained electronically and signed electronically can be treated as a Part 11 record". This is to simplify the system development perspective. As the 21 CFR Part 11 system development needs much more attention and differentiated architecture, it is important to make this call based on this definition. It's better to take a lenient approach to check Part 11 applicability, and design the system Part 11 compliant rather than a stringent check to rule it out. It's a lot harder to make it Part 11-compliant once the system is already developed.

There's a possibility to maintain a "hybrid system" as well. As the name implies, this is a combination of electronic record and paper content. Implementation of an electronic signature may become too complex for an existing system and a hybrid system may become more feasible. The electronic records can be printed and signed and the signature can be linked to the electronic record. This linking process is yet to be established and is awaiting FDA guidance. However, a procedure-based approach to ensure file name, file size, user name, etc. is sufficient.

The Part 11 assessment can be done in three stages:

1. Determine the need for Part 11 compliance
2. Determine if the system is closed or open
3. Determine if the system fulfills all the Part 11 control requirements.

Stage 1: Does Your System Need to be Part 11 Compliant?

This is a simple two-step process, shown in Figure 3.10.

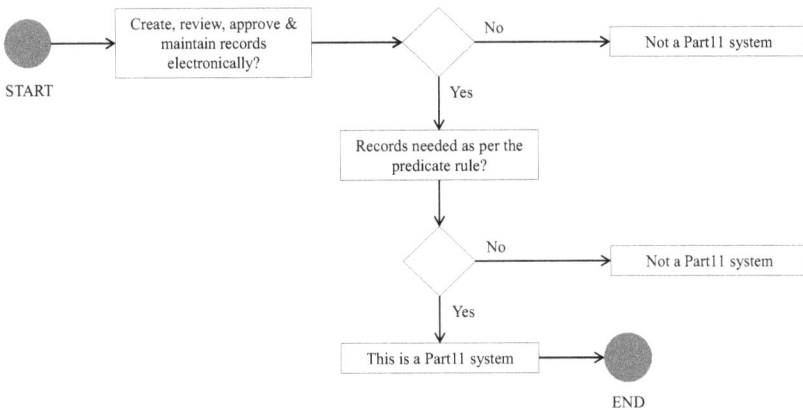

FIGURE 3.10   21 CFR Part 11 decision tree.

Stage 2: How to Know if Your System is a "Closed" or "Open" System?

A closed system means an environment in which system access is controlled by personnel who are responsible for the content of electronic records that are on the system; whereas the system access is not controlled is an open system [27]. This is an important criterion in a Part 11 system design. As an example, say you are developing a CAPA system which will have its own data entered and controlled by its users. It also needs data from an outsider, e.g. an ERP system, to get raw material information and ERP is not a Part11 compliant system. This is a combination of an open and closed system situation and special authentication needs to be applied to the raw material data to avoid contamination of CAPA data. The special authentication could be at the ERP level which can be made a closed system or data can be authenticated before transferring it to the CAPA system. The bottom-line is that the system of record, which is a Part 11 compliant system, cannot have data without being fully authenticated.

Stage 3: What Controls Should a Part 11 System Have?

The following steps provide an overview of the 21 CFR Part 11 compliance controls. This can be referred to during the system development or to check if your existing system is Part 11 compliant.

1. System delivery:
   a. The system should generate accurate and complete records
   b. Health authorities should be able to review and inspect records
2. System validation:
   a. The system needs to be validated as per the CSV process described earlier in the section
   b. All validation documents to be maintained
3. Data accuracy and integrity:
   a. The system should generate accurate and complete data
   b. The system should generate an accurate and complete report in human readable form
   c. An audit log for all activities should be done on the application to prevent data falsification
4. Records security:
   a. Authorized user access, multi-level access privileges, role-based access control
   b. No data to be accessed from outside the application
   c. Logical application security should be in place
5. System integrity:
   a. Audit log of entry, exit and every transactional activity of all users with the date and time stamp
   b. Automatic notification of illegal and failed attempts to access secure transactions
6. Audit trail:
   a. Every entry, modification, signature, tamper, re-sign of data should be audited along with the user and date time stamp
   b. No physical deletion of data. Only logical marking as "deleted" of data. The original data should be accessible
7. Signature requirements:
   a. The system should be able to display user name, date and time, reason for signature
   b. Electronic signature should be of two distinct components, such as user ID and password. This should be unique to the individual
   c. Electronic signature should never be reused
   d. Each signature should be linked with the transaction record for it not to be copied or used otherwise
8. Signature security:
   a. Entry, exit, and every transactional activity of all users into the system should be audited along with the date and time stamp
   b. Automatic notification of illegal and failed attempts to access secured transactions or fields to the responsible users

    c. The user password should not be accessible to the administrator

    d. The user password should expire after a certain time period

9. Transaction authenticity:

    a. Once a transaction has been electronically signed and authenticated, the name of the authorized person, date and time of electronic signature must be available with the transactional information. The user should give a reason for record modification

    b. The date and time change in the server to be role-specific

    c. Any signed transaction data, if changed through the application or by external means should be invalidated and be re-signed. Before the authorized person re-signs the changed transaction, it should be depicted as a tampered transaction. Automatic notification to the respective authorized user

10. Non-Repudiation:

    a. Undeniable proof of sender or receiver of data or transaction done—transactional log of all transactions along with user details, time stamp, activity description

I suggest not making the Part 11 compliant technology solution too complex by trying to implement too many controls in the system. While developing a large Part 11 system for a global central lab, we had used a data hashing mechanism to store a "data, user ID and password" combination to avoid unauthorized data modification. Any data tampering attempt or deactivating the control by the system administrator triggered an email to the Head of Quality and Head of Drug Development. We had stopped implementing technology control at this level as more controls can also be deactivated by the super administrator of the system. Hence, we had implemented a policy document, procedures, and training curricula to ensure all the users and administrator were fully aware of the requirements and agreed to follow the policy all the time. So, the combination of system, policy, procedure and training made the system work. This solution worked very well. I have tracked it for three years after the delivery of the system and found several health authority audits had no observations on the system.

This section was developed with Gurdeep S. Rooprai of Infosys. Gurdeep is an Information Technology expert and has been advising industries, including pharmaceutical companies, on technology-driven business solutions for nearly two decades.

Chapter 4

Courageous New World: Strategies to Improve Business Outcomes

The pharmaceutical industry—soon to be a trillion dollar business—is in serious trouble. Their R&D product pipeline is dry; manufacturing lacks the productivity seen in other industries, a weak supply chain causes product short-supply to worsen every year, and the marketing world is still experimenting with unfamiliar new technologies as it goes digital. Health authorities are slamming the industry with new regulations and heavy fines for non-compliance. The patient non-compliance to prescription regimen reduces the pharmaceutical sales by as much as 15%. The only silver lining is the growth in the emerging markets. How will this business survive?

This chapter discusses seven proposals to save the pharmaceutical industry in the new customer-centric world of today.

1. Staggering Genius in the Crowd: Nextgen R&D
2. Feed Your Workhorse: Smarter Manufacturing
3. Product Fast-track: Remodel the Supply Chain
4. In Digital We Trust: Industrialize Customer Centricity
5. Scream With Mouth Shut: Global Compliance Strategy
6. Why Patients Continue With Medicine: Patient Adherence
7. The Perks in Emerging Markets: Go Global

STAGGERING GENIUS IN THE CROWD: NEXTGEN R&D

I once got the opportunity to hear Sidney Taurel, Chairman of Eli Lilly, describing his vision of creating a fully integrated pharmaceutical network. Eli Lilly's R&D was evolving from fully internal lab-based experiments by their scientists using internal systems and tools, and fully funded by the company, to a network of companies, laboratories, hospitals and government facilities across the world to transform the development of drugs. This new way of working was adopted over and

Pharma's Prescription. http://dx.doi.org/10.1016/B978-0-12-407662-4.00004-0

over again by many pharmaceutical companies. A Center for Therapeutic Innovation (CTI) was established by Pfizer, the world's largest pharmaceutical company, to reinvent an open-innovation partnership model. There are several Academic Medical Centers (AMC), hospitals and universities that have partnered with Pfizer to dramatically improve R&D outcomes in this model. GlaxoSmithKline has started its open innovation laboratory, TresCantos, in Spain. They have tried to solve the very important problem of sharing intellectual properties in the open innovation world by establishing WIPO—World Intellectual Property Organization. The Novartis Institute for Biomedical Research unit was established as a separate business unit of Novartis to provide independence in decision-making and flexibility to accept help from the external world.

No other industry spends more in R&D than the pharmaceutical industry. The industry has invested over USD 500 billion in the last decade to bring in 300 products to the market but only a third of them could recover the R&D spent. There are over 5000 compounds in the pipeline in various stages of human clinical trial, but nobody would call pharmaceutical R&D a successful business. There are three major R&D issues crippling the industry—a very low success rate, a long time to market and a high cost of development. The industry needs to invent a new R&D model soon before it runs out of new drugs.

The traditional R&D model is not working and the industry has not yet found a new way of conducting R&D. Crowd sourcing, where the talents of the whole world can be utilized, can possibly be the new wave of pharmaceutical R&D. Several companies in the past have tried various ways to connect with the "crowd", but gamification was found to be one of the best ways to engage with them. It's true that not everybody likes games, but a large number of clever people do play games for several hours a day. This huge resource pool needs to be capitalized in the pharmaceutical R&D. For example, anybody can go for a USD 3 million reward in order to identify those patients who will be admitted to a hospital within the coming year using historical claims data. Or, the "crowd" can help Boehringer-Ingelheim to predict the biological response of molecules based on their chemical properties. Thousands of people have already started addressing scientific problems through computer-based games or video games. M-PMV, a 3D AIDS-causing monkey virus model, was created through a game in just 10 days by a number of players, something which had stumped scientists for 15 years [28]. This success needs to be repeated many times to make an impression on other companies making the same choice.

Pharmaceutical closed innovation is also heavily dependent on the researchers' own views that are based on scientific possibilities. This is all about the existence of diseases and the science behind curing them. This makes sense from a purely R&D perspective, creating a new IP and publishing scientific papers, but often this doesn't make business sense. So, a large part of R&D strategy should focus on looking at the existing product portfolios (within the company and competition), product differentiation possibilities and payer's opinion and also on knowing what patients want. Drugmaker AstraZeneca decided to stop development of gastrointestinal drugs as they did not think there was enough chance of developing a well-differentiated drug from the existing ones. This decision made business sense, but many R&D analysts thought the decision went against their R&D strengths as they had developed several market leaders in that therapy area. In today's industry climate, however, decisions based on business possibilities should take priority and AstraZeneca did just that.

Lately, the new pharmaceutical product launch timeline has lengthened and the cost has skyrocketed. This cost is now as high as USD 400 million for a global brand launch and often takes a very long time as launch activities start late in the product development cycle. A typical launch cost includes market research (5%), key opinion leader development (25%), marketing plan and asset development (50%) and field force activities (20%). (The percentage in parenthesis indicates the product launch cost). The R&D teams need to establish early collaboration between all the late stage stakeholders (manufacturing, marketing, sales, etc.) and improve visibility of the product's status in the development life cycle so that they can plan the launch process sooner.

An overhaul of R&D operations is long overdue. There are too many internal and external stakeholders working through complex processes. Very often we see a pharmaceutical company and a medical devices company working on the same disease but they do not communicate with each other. A combined workforce can develop the drug faster as well as keeping their own intellectual properties, as their business models do not necessarily overlap. Looking at the combined information also helps the health authorities to make a decision more quickly. Combining all parts of the life sciences industry (pharmaceutical, medical devices) can create a shared services operating model for the process areas that are not product dependent.

The industry is not ready to adopt newer technologies to harvest existing data and information that can change the way medicines are made today. The electronic medical records, patient's genetic information, genomics data and social media-based patient information need to be combined to help the physician make a better treatment decision. The treatment options are not just a decision by a physician alone—it needs to be a holistic approach. Physicians can write a more effective prescription if this information is presented in real-time. A financial filter will then be applied to narrow down the options to align with the payers. This is how new treatment options will be decided upon in the future. It is therefore not about the medicine and its values; it's about patient well-being and patient suitability that would determine the prescription. Pharmaceutical R&D need to be well aware of this trend and keep it in perspective while developing new drugs. The big data solution in cloud-based infrastructure has already made strides in the pharmaceutical R&D to assimilate data including patient data-driven analytics.

If I summarize these improvement areas to build tomorrow's R&D model, the following structure emerges (see Figure 4.1).

Open innovation, customer-driven R&D, multi-industry R&D shared services and a connected product launch are the pillars of building tomorrow's R&D of a pharmaceutical company. Many of these have been tried successfully in other industries and in pockets of pharmaceutical companies as well. But the larger benefit will only be seen with big-scale implementations.

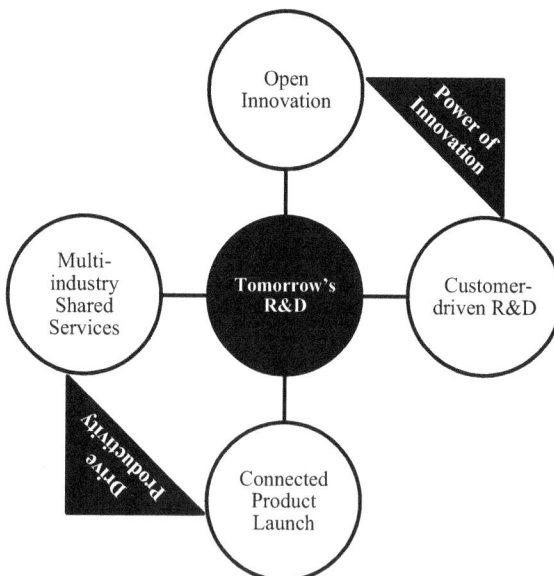

FIGURE 4.1   Tomorrow's R&D model.

My description of tomorrow's R&D has both "power of innovation" and "productivity driver". The open innovation and customer-driven R&D make the research and development more innovative, whereas multi-industry shared services and a connected product launch make R&D operations more productive, increase product speed to market and cut the operating cost drastically.

Pillar 1: Open Innovation

Proctor & Gamble had a large internal R&D set-up which was envied by the best organizations and universities worldwide who have several hundred scientists working for them. Their decision to source 50% of their desired output from external laboratories was initially shocking, but very soon became a captivating idea. So, what does a pharmaceutical company need to do to replicate this open innovation laboratory?

When I helped the head of a large biochemical and botanical R&D center to establish a long-term focus in R&D, we immediately decided to create a model which could operate under the "umbrella" of the world of open innovation. Our focus was to eliminate "closed innovation" and embrace "open innovation" by enabling people to work in a new way and to provide them with the right infrastructure. Closed innovation is the current model where all R&D activities are done within the company's own four walls. Open innovation on the other hand establishes partnerships with the leading research institutes, universities, and hospitals and also specialized small-scale scientific facilities that have very rich intellectual capital.

Open innovation strategy needs to take a top-down approach (see Figure 4.2). In my example of the large R&D center, the global head of R&D with support from the CEO made the decision to set up a new R&D center to drive open innovation. The strategy was to define compound needs internally in collaboration with the sales and marketing teams, but get the right external laboratories on board to develop those compounds. We had also planned to create an internal infrastructure

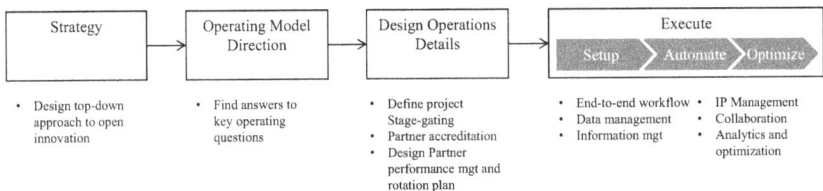

FIGURE 4.2   Open innovation model.

to receive and maintain intellectual assets, data, information and the entire knowledge base of compounds. The strategy also highlighted the need for project stage-gating to make financial and project continuation decisions.

After the strategy development, we encountered several challenges working with the various R&D stakeholders as they had many questions in embarking on this journey for the first time. Several key questions were dealt with and answered in the next phase—the "operating model direction" of the program.

Management teams. What capabilities do we develop to meet R&D goals? How do we ensure the right balance between the internal and external resources? How do I monitor and track all the projects effectively, including those that are being executed externally?

Operations strategy. How do I select partners, measure success or failure and rotate partners? How do I measure project success or failures and make go/no-go decisions? How do I align all the projects upfront to the project stage-gating process?

Legal/Finance. How do we assign IP rights to the jointly developed intellectual properties?

Operations teams. How do I get data and information from the collaborators in real-time? How do I ensure I don't just get the abstract level information or derived conclusions, and that I have access to the raw data for my own assessments? How do I standardize dataset for all the partners to eliminate data issues when they return them?

Regulatory submissions. How do I get project visibility upfront to plan the regulatory submissions on time?

External partners. How do I get access to systems/data/people to collaborate work across firewalls?

Answers to some of these questions led us to "design operations details" to create processes, methods and implementation tools that would help establish operations more effectively.

Stage-gating a research project at various milestones is an important design parameter for open innovation success. We designed a stage-gating framework which is described in Figure 4.3.

The most important design principle in open innovation is the approach to external partnerships. The development of a strong partner accreditation program needs to begin early in the program. It is well understood that the accreditation program is never going to be perfect, but it's an ongoing effort to get to the highest maturity level. Internal as

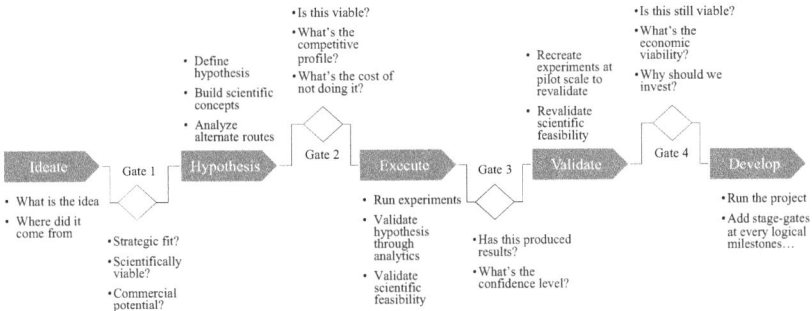

FIGURE 4.3   Innovation stage-gating framework.

well as external stakeholders will need to go through a continual learning process throughout the entire partnership process.

The accreditation process we had built for this R&D set-up consisted of strategic fitment criteria design, creation of an advisory council to nominate partners, partner onboarding, training, certification, scorecards and reports, and a collaboration framework to make the partnership work.

The advisory council was given a guideline to recommend a partner. The potential partner should have the following:

- An ability to meet all the research needs as well as local regulatory and legal compliance requirements
- An ability to adopt to the company work culture and align with the strategic thinking
- An ability to bring in innovative ideas to enhance the internal R&D values of the company
- An ability to work independently with the existing lab infrastructure
- Proven track record of meeting these criteria over time
- Any other criteria—the parameters need to be adjusted to meet specific partnership situations and also for a specific project.

The partnership can also be classified based on the level of services a partner would provide. A partner with capabilities to support a project independently with their people, lab, and other facilities will be the "category-1" partner. A smaller lab with niche skills without much infrastructure may become the "category-4" partner, whereas "category-2" and "category-3" can be created in between. The partner onboarding process and level of training and scorecarding on their performance will depend on their partnership category level. This is very important to make an apples to apples comparison when it comes to the performance evaluation of partners.

Pillar 2: Customer-Driven R&D

In today's world, customer-driven R&D is imperative for a successful product development and launch. Several product companies have created a consumer council to receive product feedback, challenges and ideas to expand the product. This council includes not only the company's existing customers or potential customers, but also the customers of other product companies including those of competitors.

Pharmaceutical companies have always been more focused on the scientific possibilities of product improvement or the development of new products. This shows the ability of basic research to introduce a new product for a therapy but most of the time it does not meet economic criteria. While working on "lab to plant process scale-up" unit, I have seen several processes get rejected as they were not initially designed for a commercial scale operation. This shows that the scientific community's heart lies in innovative product development and does not necessarily focus on the product economies. This mindset needs to change and when that happens, I'm sure scientists will open up more to ideas from their customers. I have numerous experiences in attending physician conventions that are dominated by the marketing and sales teams; the legal and finance teams also attend as monitors. However, this is a golden opportunity missed by the R&D community to hear the physicians talk about the products they have developed. The product adverse event reports, signal detection and product complaints are not only used to complete the regulatory process, but can also be used to learn about product improvement opportunities.

The need for aligning R&D teams to the customers, similar to the way sales and marketing teams do, is eminent for R&D productivity improvement. The physicians, patients, payers, providers, university medical centers and caregivers can contribute significantly to the R&D pipeline and improve existing products. I'm confident that health authorities will be flexible enough to support R&D innovations by modifying regulatory requirements, if this improves healthcare significantly.

Pillar 3: Multi-Industry Shared Services

My definition of multi-industry here is not really to connect disjointed industries through shared services. It is to connect pharmaceutical industries with medical devices or biotechnology companies, who all independently develop and market products for the same disease areas. There are significant opportunities to reduce the timeline, eliminate duplications and reduce the cost multifold, if some of the development activities are carried out together. There are several common stakeholder groups and services such as product analysis, compound screening, trial management, project management, data management, data analysis, reporting, sample management, clinical supply management, patient recruitment, result analysis, etc. are done by many different stakeholders, such as sponsor companies, CROs, IT companies, consulting organizations and hospitals. They are done in isolation, repeatedly, generating duplicate data and information that are not always independently helpful. Individually they may pick up some hypothesis which has already been proven wrong by others and which can be avoided by sharing information between stakeholders. There is a better solution to connect stakeholders.

When I advised a global clinical research organization (CRO) to streamline their global trial management processes and build a single system to support all the processes globally, it sounded like an uphill task for all of us (see Figure 4.4). However, when the solution was successfully delivered almost 18 months later, we all celebrated this great achievement. We had consolidated all the activities needed for the IND stage through to the NDA stage including regulatory submission document creation. We had then looked at all the stakeholders involved to execute those activities and the systems and tools that were used in the end to end workflow. There were opportunities including simplification of processes, stakeholder interactions, systems integrations and automation of several manual processes. We all agreed—consultants and the CRO stakeholders—to create a new model for clinical trial operations. The idea was to eliminate manual touch points for sample kit distribution, subject enrollment, sample collections, analysis report assembly and follow-up with the investigators for result interpretations, etc. We

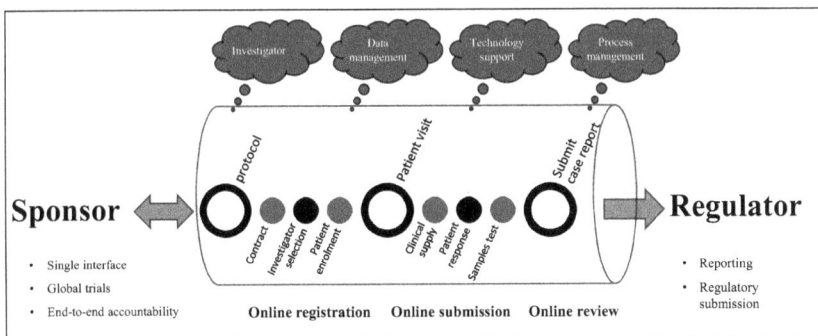

FIGURE 4.4   Drug development in a box.

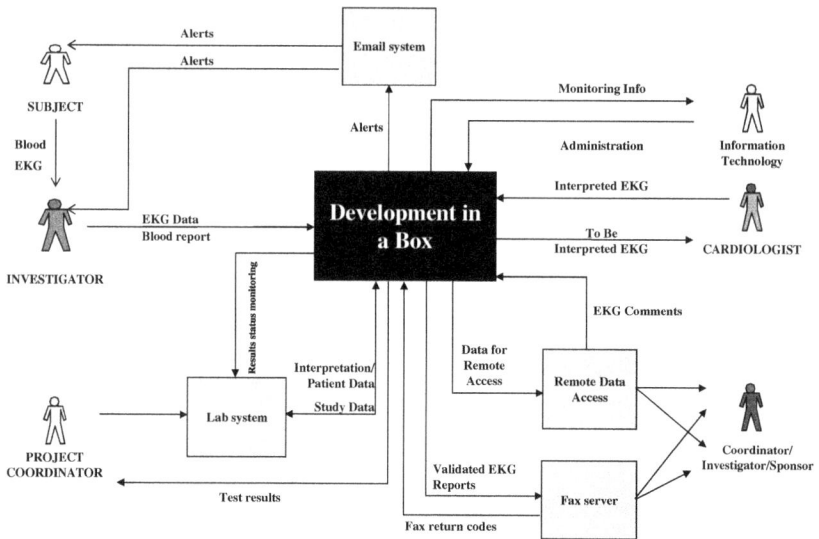

FIGURE 4.5   Drug development in a box use case.

had designed a technology platform which could manage these activities end to end without moving samples and papers to multiple locations.

The diagram in Figure 4.5 is one of the many use cases that were automated through the "drug development in a box" platform. This use case is for a subject going to her family physician after completing all clinical trial enrolment formalities online. Through company training, her physician could access the system to understand the entire process and the analysis needs. The physician collected a blood sample and sent it for analysis; she did an EKG as defined in the protocol. When results were available, the physician uploaded them into the "drug development in a box" portal. The EKG result was sent online to the cardiologist for interpretation. The entire process was available in the system for the sponsor or project coordinator to monitor, track and take appropriate action.

The data generated in this platform was always as per the standard defined upfront, which eliminated data standardization issues encountered in most of the clinical trials. Analytics were done and refreshed as and when data flowed in—there were no dependencies on the data management teams to update data, cleanse data or inform the analytics team to run reports. The regulatory submissions teams were aware of the data availability to get ready well in advance for the submission documents. The entire process operated in a streamlined way and created standard data which was visible to all the relevant stakeholders who could analyze the data for early failure of the compound, in order to save time and money.

With the private Cloud options available now, it has improved even more. It will now be the future of clinical trial execution and management.

The above example is to bring in several stakeholders to work in a shared environment without impacting on the others' routine jobs. The shared services help to consolidate activities that are repetitive in nature and aren't dependent on any specific therapeutic area.

With technology advancement in R&D operations, there is a significant amount of work that has become very routine while many other tasks require special scientific knowledge and training [29]. A thorough analysis of R&D activities could easily differentiate these two different activity types. The routine work can be executed through a shared pool of people to drive productivity improvement by reducing silos, eliminating redundancies and providing effective knowledge management. This shared services model has three components—(1) activities that require Therapeutic Area (TA) knowledge; (2) work that can be done in a shared services model but that is highly dependent on activities described under (1) above; and (3) the activities that are routine and can be executed independently (See Figure 4.6). The TA aligned work and TA dependent activities need to be co-located; however, the independent shared services activities can be done from a low cost location to drive down the operating cost.

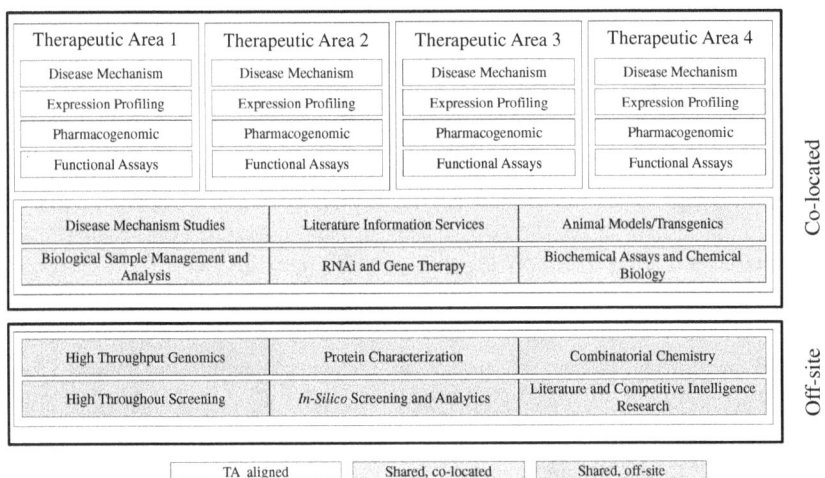

FIGURE 4.6   R&D activity grouping.

Some of these activities are common even with the larger stakeholders, e.g. medical devices. So, once the shared services are well established within a pharmaceutical company, this can even be extended to medical devices organizations to increase the benefits further.

Pillar 4: Connected Product Launch

The new product launch is a very involved process and takes time and money to get right. A product doesn't just sell on its benefit and safety information unless communicated to the customers effectively. This is done through the product launch process. The product launch is important and its effectiveness can easily differentiate it from the peer group.

Today's new product launch is costly and takes longer than it should. The prime cause of the problem is not creating early visibility of the product status to all the stakeholders involved in the launch process. This was very clear when I helped a top pharmaceutical company in Europe. The problem was well understood by the senior leadership teams globally and they decided to bring in a technology-enabled process to connect all the stakeholders in a product launch right at the beginning of the drug development process. This resulted in a big improvement in new product launch speed and sharing a knowledge base across various countries globally. While I can't disclose the exact strategy to launch this global brand efficiently, here are some details of the solution which can be replicated.

Our initial analysis found several problem areas, including: (a) a long product launch cycle with inconsistent launch packets; (b) no or minimum visibility of the new product pipeline amongst stakeholders—research, development, clinical manufacturing, early stage marketing and late stage sales teams; (c) usage of obsolete product documents by sales teams were common practice; and (d) an inconsistent process, information and structure in different brand teams, and in different geographies. The result was high cost, slow product launches and (e) they all had their own tools to manage product information.

We designed a product launch portal which established a collaborative work environment for all the stakeholders (see Figure 4.7). Stakeholder mapping ensured all teams were connected all the time. They each had a specific workspace to work on their part of the product content and share it with others as needed. The entire team got the visibility of the current status of the product development on a real-time basis. The portal also had the ability to integrate with the content creation systems

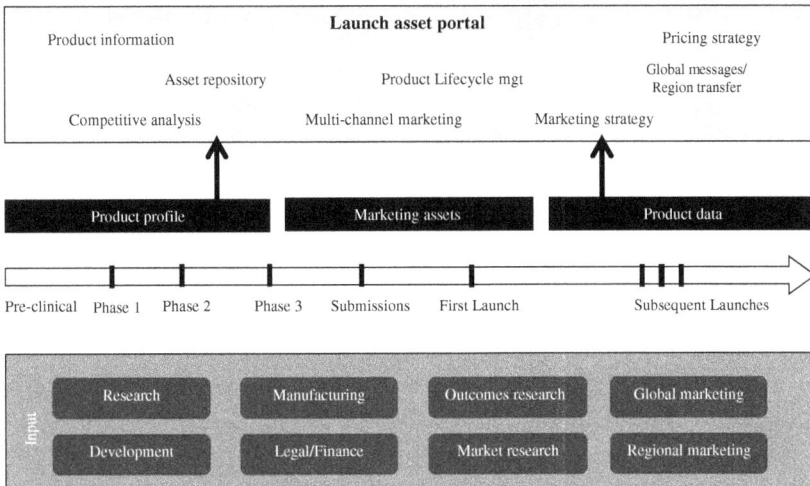

FIGURE 4.7   Connected product launch.

to seamlessly track the availability of marketing content for the launch. The company had created significant benefits through this program:

- Reduction in product launch cycletime up to 40%
- Sales and marketers were enabled with the latest product marketing assets throughout the entire asset life cycle
- A clearly defined launch life cycle, process, roles, hand-off requirements. All were connected through a single system to eliminate errors
- Seamless transition between teams. Hand-off between global and regional marketers for uniform messaging. Standardized hand-off kits for all products shared between teams
- A single source of accurate information. No need to enter into multiple systems for product information.

The solution was a huge success at all stakeholder levels. The initial change management took a while but the value created by the solution was self explanatory to move into the new ways of working.

Now is the time to re-evaluate R&D operations at all companies. Improvement opportunities are countless and very similar amongst many R&D teams. Good news is that there are examples of process, organization and technology-driven R&D innovations and productivity improvements that can be scaled up to create a greater pharmaceutical industry impact. These solutions have already been proven to reduce the drug development timeline and increase predictability early enough to cut development cost.

FEED YOUR WORKHORSE: SMARTER MANUFACTURING

Imagine if you could mix a few ingredients yourself in your study room to make the medicine you want. You have just printed all the ingredients needed using your 3D printer to make your medicines as prescribed by your physician. This is no more cumbersome than making a tall latte in the kitchen. This may happen soon—technology is being invented fast.

Until 3D printing or something similar becomes part of our household gadgets, an alternate option is also possible. This is to eliminate some formulations, packaging, storing and retailer services, and send product raw materials directly to the patients or caregivers who can prepare the final form themselves (see Figure 4.8). This will reduce the cost of the drug to one thousandth.

The prime reasons for product formulation is to make a dosage form which a patient can administer directly, which can deliver the active ingredients to the target action area within the body and help to release the product appropriately and preserve the active ingredients for longer. The packaging helps with the distribution and long-term storage of the product. While we all enjoy the final form of the medicine which we can use directly, it comes with a huge price tag attached to it. Will a patient who is not in acute care but in chronic care, preventive care or taking lifestyle drugs take the option of buying medicine at one thousandth of the price? I believe so. The active ingredient cost of many popular drugs in the United States and their retail prices were reported by the US department of commerce in their "true cost of your prescription drugs" study. While this study was widely disputed, the report gives us a view of the cost of the active ingredient which is responsible for our wellness and the actual price we pay. A couple of examples from the report are: the cost of Celecoxib, the active ingredient of the brand Celebrex, is 61 cents while the retail price of a 100 mg tablet in a 100 tablet pack is USD 130.27; the active ingredient of the brand Claritin costs only 71 cents, whereas a

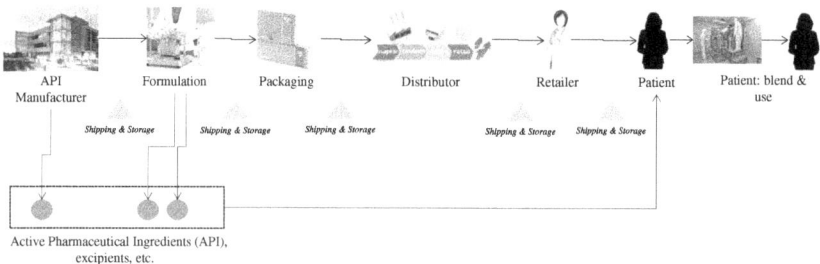

FIGURE 4.8   Smarter manufacturing.

Claritin 100 mg tablet in a 100 tablet pack costs USD 215.17 [30]. Let me ask the question again—will you want to buy your medicine at 61 cents plus USD 5 shipping and handling, which will then take 15 minutes of your time to prepare the final form before you can swallow it, or do you want to pay USD 130.27 for the same medicine which you can swallow directly? I definitely see a unanimous yes to the former option. The price difference between the active ingredient and a generic product is not as high as the branded product, but there's still a huge difference.

I have spent several years in pharmaceutical manufacturing and was very intrigued by this fact, and also very excited to advocate the consumer-driven manufacturing option. If I were in a manufacturing plant today, I would have started a pilot by now. I'm sure many of you will do so soon. The whole idea is to manufacture the active ingredient, milling them to an extent which can be used by a patient and is easy to mix with the excipient or coating agent, if needed. As the mixing of the active ingredient, excipient and any other substance needed for targeted delivery or controlled dissolution of the active ingredient inside the body will be done by the patients themselves at home, the product needs to be sent in a form which will be easy to handle by the patient or a caregiver.

Some of the current processes are left for the formulation unit simply because it's part of today's way of working. The milling, blending and small-scale packing can be done in an Active Pharmaceutical Ingredient (API) manufacturing plant set-up to further reduce the cost of running a formulation plant.

The whole process will work like this. A patient will order the medicine or a caregiver will do the same on behalf of a patient to a manufacturing company or their authorized agents. The pharmaceutical manufacturer will dispense materials including active ingredients, excipients, binders, etc. as per the prescription and the formulation recipe. They will directly ship everything to the mailing address of the caregiver or the patient. There's no shipment and storage hold-up at the formulation plant, distributors and retailers—the product reaches the patient directly. The patient needs to use some tools (I assume the pharmaceutical equipment manufacturers will make some equipment for home use) or they can use a simple mortar and pestle to mix the products as instructed by the manufacturer before using them. Depending on the product's heat sensitivity, stability and safety, patients can make a bulk quantity or make and consume small quantities daily.

I know I have oversimplified this, but this is a definite possibility. I would recommend taking a no-risk approach and start with the OTC products. It sounds very outdated to be told to use old-fashioned techniques when we are used to a very different lifestyle. However, we are at a juncture where technology sophistication is taking us back in time to a simpler life where we could get things done at home at a very affordable price. Think about IKEA and how they have changed the concept of buying household furniture. You buy a chair but you take home a few wooden blocks in a small packet which is easy to carry. You spend 15 minutes of your time to assemble them. Now you can even increase your sense of pride by claiming yourself to be a carpenter who has built a wooden chair by himself. The Home Depot has said it all in their slogan: "You Can Do It. We Can Help". I understand you must be thinking how crazy I am to compare furniture assembly with medicine preparation, but this is just a logical comparison to show the world of possibilities. The formulation processes are not very tricky—they can be handled on a very small scale which can be managed by all of us. I do also understand the serious argument about safety issues around handling active ingredients at home. There are several possibilities: (a) it is dispensed at a very small quantity anyway and it may not be as hazardous as handling a large amount; (b) the patient handles it in a disposable contained area with gloves and masks supplied with the shipment as a "tools and accessories kit", just like the small tools you get with IKEA products; and (c) restrict this possibility for dangerous goods.

I would definitely want to give it a try. I want to give it a try because this is smarter manufacturing. I see this as making the consumer more powerful in controlling the price of medicine themselves as opposed to getting trapped in the maze of insurance companies, provider, manufacturer and physician. And this will free up a large amount of money from the healthcare spend we have today.

In line with smarter cities coming up with smarter homes, I can certainly envisage a medicine preparation cabinet with a sterilization facility, air purification system and an air exhaust unit that will facilitate formulating our own medicine.

Let's look at some of the financial statistics to make this medicine unit at home. The prescription drug spend in the US in 2012 was USD 325.7 billion. If I assume that 50% of medicines are easy to use with no special technique needed to formulate the dosage forms, the potential reduction opportunity is USD 165 billion. If the math is correct, the industry will be able to take out about 60% of the cost of prescription drugs which will be close to USD 100 billion. This is enough to fund more than 50 new drugs to market every year. This is a huge opportunity for pharmaceutical manufacturing which should not be missed.

Now, let's make our API manufacturing units smarter too. Patients will very soon start complaining that the 61 cents they pay for the active ingredient is too high and that it should be reduced further. The manufacturing plants have the opportunity for productivity driven cost optimization.

The blockbuster drug era is over for the pharmaceutical industry. This will impact on the manufacturing production planning to make products in smaller batches. This goes well with my recommendation of re-designing pharmaceutical companies to make them smaller and more nimble. The manufacturing production units will follow suit.

The workhorse of manufacturing is flanked by two overstressed functions—R&D and Sales & Marketing in the pharmaceutical value chain. Unlike R&D and Sales & Marketing, manufacturing issues do not create industry-wide turbulence as it mainly deals with the company's internal stakeholders. While R&D challenges or sales problems are on "burning platforms", manufacturing issues also need attention.

For manufacturing operations, it's mandatory not to deviate from any steps defined in the approved recipe for a product. At the same time, manufacturing needs to be more productive, efficient, and deliver higher throughput to make it a low cost operation without compromising on quality. Typical manufacturing costs are around 35% of sales, but this varies widely for branded drugs and generics. The generic COGS (Cost of Goods Sold) has a much higher ratio with the sales in comparison to branded drugs. As McKinsey reports, the potential productivity-driven improvement can reduce the cost of pharmaceutical manufacturing by USD 50 billion [31].

Pharma manufacturing is capital and labor intensive; over 90% of the cost is for the raw materials, utilities and human resources. All of these could be optimized enough to improve the horse-power of the workhorse. Also the average capacity utilization of pharmaceutical plants is just around 30–40% [32]. Work is typically done in silos with multiple stakeholders having divergent, at times even competitive drivers. Production, for example, would work to ensure an increase in productivity, whereas Environmental Health & Safety (EH&S) would push them to ensure minimal environmental impact and the safety of the employees, even if that implies a decrease in productivity. So, the combination of improving labor productivity, reducing variable costs, improving plant utilization and better collaboration between stakeholders can make the manufacturing plants more productive. The diagram in Figure 4.9 is a representation of some of the improvement areas for various stakeholders.

From my many years of experience working in pharmaceutical manufacturing plants, both as a doer and a consultant, I found that the stakeholders were not identifying improvement opportunities or setting a goal to make things possible. Goal setting and achieving are nicely

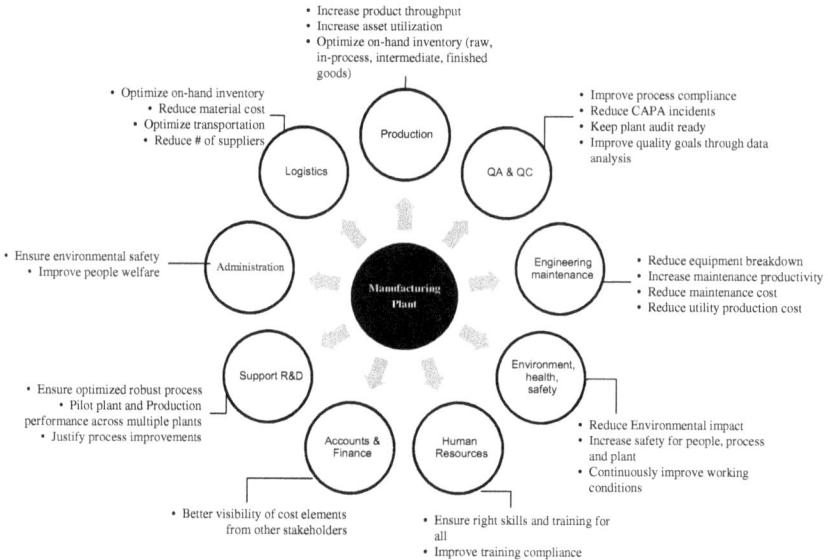

FIGURE 4.9   Manufacturing improvement opportunities.

implemented for sales, marketing and even in R&D organizations but
rarely done in manufacturing operations. Here I refer to the improvement goals and not routine goals such as production quantity, schedule,
inventory and quality. When I worked in a small production unit manufacturing oncology products on a smaller scale because of their higher
price, I was more successful in implementing improvement goals than
while running larger production units with many moving parts. We used
some of the following elements to improve plant productivity:

Design a shop-floor learning management solution. Production
productivity is largely dependent on the empowering of production
engineers, supervisors and shop-floor managers through enhanced
product knowledge. This is not always about giving them the authority to act but rather to improve their product and process knowledge
to make better decisions.
Improve plant design. Pharmaceutical manufacturing history is very
old, but we are still using many methods and systems that have been
around for centuries. Modern plant design can make the operations
more productive.
Improve information management and stakeholder collaboration.
Effective information management can enable manufacturing functions to make analytics-based decision-making; it also increases
visibility to all the stakeholders.

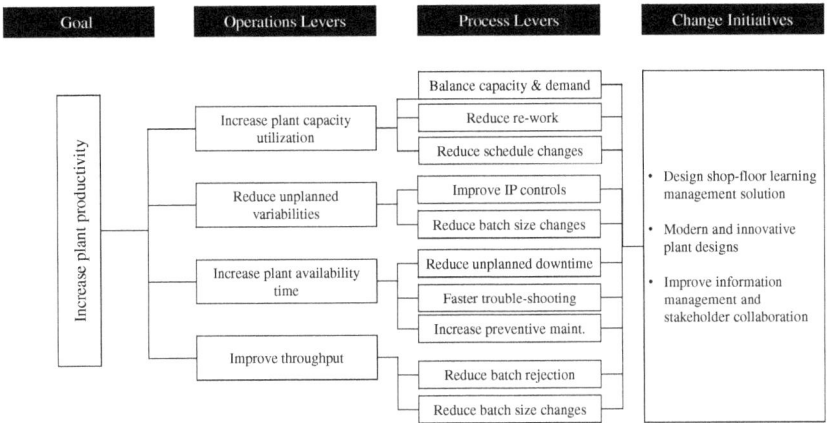

FIGURE 4.10   Manufacturing value diagram.

I have derived several improvement opportunities or change initiatives from a structured analysis of the manufacturing goals (see the diagram in Figure 4.10).

The shop-floor learning management system is the best mechanism to solve manufacturing process issues quickly and effectively. While working on the shop floor I came across several situations when a quick and the right decision could recover a production batch from failure. These batches are worth millions and the production manager and all of the crew will do their best to not destroy the product. However, if they do not get the additional support they need from R&D or other teams, either because it happened on an early morning shift or the right people were not available to help, shop-floor teams fail to do much. A learning management system with production information, R&D information and Q&A sessions on possible "what if" scenarios, a history of failures with recommended solutions, and a document library can make the shop-floor team much more powerful in recovering a production batch (see Figure 4.11).

The analytics component of this system can provide a significant insight into the issues of the various plant stakeholders. Some signs can be an early warning of a larger problem. While working on a night shift I found the steam consumption of a production batch was much higher than the limit of a normal batch. I called the boiler operator to double check the records in the boiler house and he confirmed the high consumption of steam in the in-process batch. I ran out of the process control room to alert the reactor supervisor about the possible failure of the reactor temperature control system. It was reading the temperature incorrectly and the steam control valve did not close enough to stop the steam

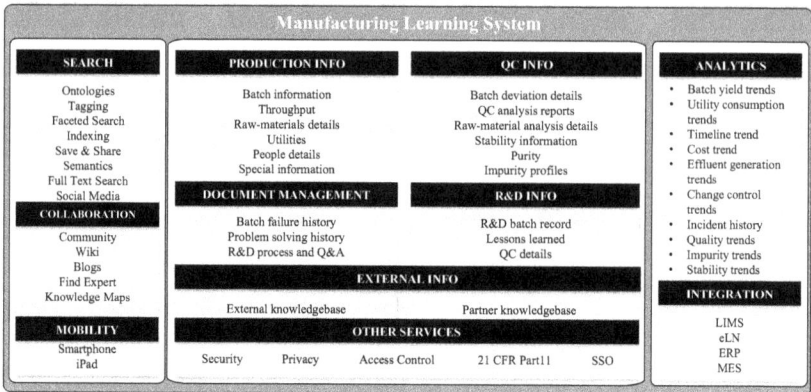

Manufacturing Learning System			
SEARCH	**PRODUCTION INFO**	**QC INFO**	**ANALYTICS**
Ontologies Tagging Faceted Search Indexing Save & Share Semantics Full Text Search Social Media	Batch information Throughput Raw-materials details Utilities People details Special information	Batch deviation details QC analysis reports Raw-material analysis details Stability information Purity Impurity profiles	• Batch yield trends • Utility consumption trends • Timeline trend • Cost trend • Effluent generation trends • Change control trends • Incident history • Quality trends • Impurity trends • Stability trends
COLLABORATION	**DOCUMENT MANAGEMENT**	**R&D INFO**	
Community Wiki Blogs Find Expert Knowledge Maps	Batch failure history Problem solving history R&D process and Q&A	R&D batch record Lessons learned QC details	
	EXTERNAL INFO		**INTEGRATION**
	External knowledgebase	Partner knowledgebase	LIMS eLN
MOBILITY	**OTHER SERVICES**		ERP MES
Smartphone iPad	Security Privacy Access Control 21 CFR Part11 SSO		

FIGURE 4.11 Manufacturing shop-floor learning model.

supply. Without knowing how long this had been happening I could sense a major problem with the product as the reaction continued at a much higher temperature than standard. I stopped the steam supply manually and checked the reaction completion which was done by the time we noticed the temperature problem—the high temperature had accelerated the reaction and it was completed faster. In any case, I decided to move on to the next stage of the process with additional in-process QC checks. We were lucky and the product was saved with some loss of yield, but that's a different story. It was only possible because we had a fully integrated plant with many of its system parameters visible to the production managers. If it had been a disjoined operation with no trend data available, we would not have been able to find the fault and would have lost the batch completely. It could have been worse and resulted in a major accident if the temperature had shot up too high. This was a good example of having integrated data analytics and collaboration between teams to improve manufacturing productivity.

One of the major issues in production is to clean equipment between batches. With high production schedules the cleaning operation becomes a bottleneck, especially if there's a product switch in the assembly line. Though most of the latest manufacturing units come with CIP (Cleaning in Place), the batch delay may still occur. The cleaning, cleanse analysis, sterilization, validation, etc. take a lot of time between the batches. Modern design technique should consider using disposable containers instead of reusable production assembly. This is feasible for smaller size batches with small gaps between two batches and will be necessary for smaller production dispatches as in those for orphan drugs and personalized medicines. Millipore has already introduced single-use bioreactor systems for mammalian cell culture, delivering several of these benefits [33]. I welcome their innovation.

Smarter manufacturing will transform pharmaceutical manufacturing operations soon. They will be more customer centric and will adapt to the work model in many other industries such as Retail and Consumer Products. The move is essential to save the industry.

PRODUCT FAST-TRACK: REMODEL THE SUPPLY CHAIN

Irrespective of age, gender or location, all of us have been to drug stores for medicines—most of the time for a simple medicine to treat a cold and at other more unfortunate times for prescription drugs.

It is no different for Sheila, a resident of Naples, Florida. She comes to the local drug store to fill the prescription for her aged mother. But the medicine is out of stock. She is surprised to learn that the manufacturer of the medicine she needs operates from a neighboring state and is still unable to maintain the stock. The supply chain of this medicine does not work.

Sheila is unhappy—she has three options. She goes to another store to buy the same brand and the retailer loses the business. Sheila may agree to an alternate brand which will mean the product manufacturer loses the business. Or, she might decide not to buy the medicine for now and leave both the retailer and manufacturer empty-handed. The latter decision can put an even greater burden on the US healthcare system if her mother needs hospitalization for not complying with the medication. All these issues can be eliminated through a well-planned supply chain execution solution.

This example shows how product non-availability directly impacts on a company's revenue. Supply chain capabilities need to be robust enough for continuous delivery on time and at the right places to make the product available to the customers. The end to end supply chain model in the pharmaceutical industry needs to be tightened up to withstand existing and upcoming pressures. The supply chain model covers the entire range of processes from development of the drug through making it available on the store shelves to finding its way into the patients' cabinets. This also ensures effective product recall if required.

However, the supply chain mechanism in the pharmaceutical industry is complex. Too many manufacturers, distributors, retailers and several product import and export dynamics make the supply chain more complicated. The situation is different in the mature markets as opposed to the emerging markets. India has over 20,000 pharmaceutical manufacturers, 60,000 distributors and over 750,000 retailers which make the supply chain very complex. The US imports 80% of their active pharmaceutical ingredients and over 40% of their finished products from foreign countries. This puts extra pressure on the supply chain system.

In the fall of last year, there were 55 deaths because of contaminated drug use in the US. There are similar reports across various countries around the world. A regulation to track and trace products will soon be implemented to remove adulterated drugs from the system, but it may put additional pressure on the supply chain.

US healthcare reform has shifted its focus from the product to the patient. This will have an impact on the current product-centric supply chain to evolve into a consumer-centric model.

While the current supply chain has improvement opportunities and there are several upcoming challenges, this is under cost pressure too. The pharmaceutical supply chain is oscillating between value additions and cost savings. The supply chain typically accounts for about 50% of the costs, 40% of the headcount and 60% of the capital of a large pharmaceutical firm. So there are obvious areas for productivity improvements and cost savings that can free up money very quickly. As a result, the supply chain executives are under pressure to drive down the cost and put it at the top of the agenda. However, in the new world of volatile demand, shorter product life cycles and stringent regulatory control, the focus on cost savings alone will not help to transform the supply chain system.

The journey towards transforming the supply chain needs to start with a focus on maximizing value while keeping an eye on cost control. Business executives understand the value dimension but show an ambivalent position towards value definition, tracking and delivering it through the supply chain network. From my varied experience of pharmaceutical supply chain strategy. We can see a clear trend in the lack of collaboration between all the supply chain stakeholders within the organization. This makes supply chain planning very weak and mostly fails to deliver value. Other related issues are not having joint planning, insufficient planning details and taking quick actions based on monitoring reports.

5-5-5 Model: Connected Supply Chain

We have introduced the connected supply chain model (see Figure 4.12) to ensure the right strategy, execution planning, review, implementation and control of the supply chain solution to drive value to a company and to its customers. This model, which we have named the 5-5-5 Model, ensures the right strategy-driven supply chain management. The Model connects five strategic, five planning and five implementation elements to create an end to end model.

5-5-5 Model: Connected Supply Chain

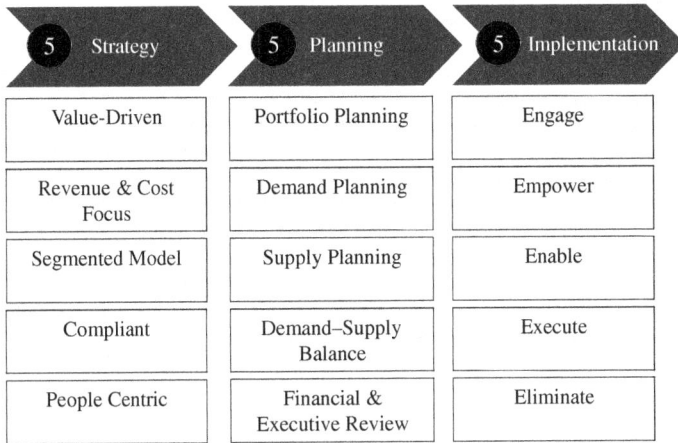

5 Strategy	5 Planning	5 Implementation
Value-Driven	Portfolio Planning	Engage
Revenue & Cost Focus	Demand Planning	Empower
Segmented Model	Supply Planning	Enable
Compliant	Demand–Supply Balance	Execute
People Centric	Financial & Executive Review	Eliminate

FIGURE 4.12   Connected Supply Chain.

Strategy

The supply chain-driven values are well articulated both for the external stakeholders as well as internal. The key external values include on-time product availability to customers and the elimination of drug short supply. Another value to customers would be passing on the cost savings in the reduction of the medicine price so that consumers can get better value for money.

Value Driven. The value to the company or shareholder comes from the supply chain improvement initiatives. Shareholder values can be defined in terms of free cash flow which is impacted through the revenue and cost balancing.

Supply chain transformation initiatives need to look at value creation opportunities not only within their own organization but also with trading partners such as suppliers, distributors and customers. With technological advancement, especially in the areas of business intelligence and collaboration, it is easier than ever to define and measure these value creation opportunities.

Revenue and Cost Focus. The supply chain can contribute to improving the revenue by doing a simple task—supplying the right product at the right time, at the right place and in the right quantity. An optimized supply chain can also improve the drug development speed by delivering clinical supply materials efficiently. It can also help introduce a new product to the market more quickly.

Reduce cost. The supply chain cost is significant in the overall cost of a company. An efficient supply chain can reduce the cost by reducing the finished goods and in-process product inventories, reducing raw materials stocks, optimizing the warehouse and reducing transportation costs.

Reduce working capital needs. Most of the supply chains have already developed capabilities around inventory optimization but they also need to look at how accounts receivable and accounts payable processes can be improved as these contribute to working capital as well.

Reduce effective tax rates. Several countries outside the US and several states within the US have preferential tax treatments for different investment types. While making decisions about the supply chain network, these tax benefits must be considered.

Segmented Model. The traditional supply chain approach of "one size fits all" will not be able to deliver the values and cost promises that are expected from this function. Products in a pharmaceutical company can be segmented by their therapeutic areas such as primary care, specialty and oncology. There are several product types within each therapy area—some are new and some have had a steady market for a while. Some products have a constant market demand, whereas some are very unstable. The supply chain capabilities for each of these products may be different. The 5-5-5 model differentiates these various capabilities through the "Supply Chain Segmentation" (see Figure 4.13).

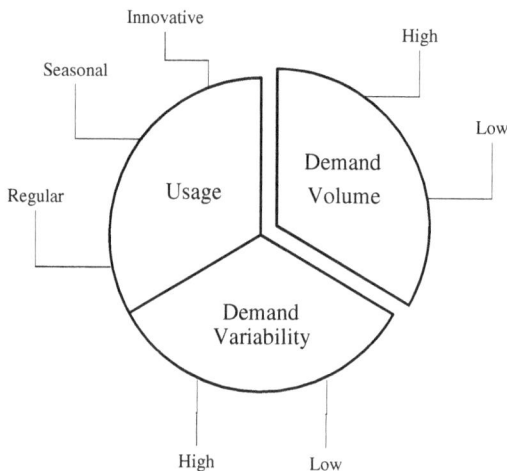

FIGURE 4.13 Supply Chain segmentation.

We recommend different supply chain designs based on the following segmentation parameters:

- Usage pattern/Product types—regular, seasonal, innovative
- Demand volume—high, low
- Demand variability—high, low.

Based on the segmentation, the supply chain capabilities may need to change. For example, products that are characterized by high volume and low variability will need an efficient supply chain where the focus needs to be on relentless execution. This type of supply chain is often characterized by a predictable demand and supply variability, and a reliable and high volume supply chain. Existing supply chain processes and systems may be sufficient for this type of product supply chain with an increased focus on efficiency. Technology-driven optimization of supply network, transportation and manufacturing can make a big difference.

For products that are in an innovation category, the supply chain needs to be nimble. Most of the time these products have very high variability on the demand side and often on the supply side as well. An organization with innovative products needs to develop capabilities on a predictive supply chain model. This model should be able to sense demand and create enough agility in the supply network to react to any changes in demand and supply situations quickly.

Compliance Focus. The compliance requirements in the pharmaceutical industry are changing rapidly and the supply chain is also affected. One such regulatory mandate is on its way—Product track & trace. The track & trace capability will allow organizations to have complete control over the movement of goods to respond to any risky events in the supply chain by developing capabilities to:

- Track any product on the market which is claimed as your product but isn't. Track down counterfeit drugs
- Track goods at production sites, including CMOs or third-party packaging sites
- Know exactly which drug from which batch needs to be recalled or what has expired
- Pinpoint exactly which pharmacies, hospitals, or stores end up with tainted products on their shelves.

Regulators are raising the bar on supply chain safety, demanding sophisticated technology solutions to track and trace products from raw materials to patient use. As estimated by the Center for Medicines in the Public Interest (2010) the global sale of counterfeit drugs would reach

USD 75 billion, which is a 92% increase in just five years. Today, many governments require supply chain participants to maintain chain-of-custody records that prove the origin and authenticity of each product. Item-level serialization and track and trace capabilities enable better supply chain visibility which can challenge the counterfeiters and improve business performance. The FDA has said it plans to issue draft guidance in 2013 on standards for track and trace of prescription drug packages, intended to help secure the supply chain on a national standard. The California e-Pedigree law is likely to come into effect by 2015 and will require significant effort on the side of pharmaceutical companies to comply with this law [34]. For example:

- Generic and brand manufacturers must comply with e-Pedigree for 50% of their products by 2015 and the remaining 50% by 2016. (Percentages can be based on unit volume, SKU, or drug product family.)
- Wholesalers and re-packagers must comply with e-Pedigree by July 2016
- Pharmacies and pharmacy warehouses must comply with e-Pedigree by July 2017.

People Centric. The people aspect of the supply chain is often ignored in the supply chain strategy. The supply chain is a people-dependent function and the execution falls flat without having the right people on the job to execute the strategy. One of the key people aspects is to enable stakeholders to embrace into the new way of working. They may need to change at various levels to make the strategy work. The details are discussed in the implementation section.

Planning

There are different planning processes in an organization—planning for new products, demand planning, supply planning, financial planning and strategic planning. All these are currently being performed at different maturity levels. The reasons for not reaching the highest level of maturity are the differences in functional mandates, processes, departmental styles and people who work there. Most of these planning processes are dependent on each other. Given that the pharmaceutical product portfolio is complex and that they operate in many silos, the most important need is to bring all stakeholders into a single plan which is signed off by everyone. Are you kidding? This is just like selling the world. But the truth is that more and more disjointed functions need to come together to operate through a single plan or at least be aligned with each other. This is a fundamental shift from the current practice of working through several functional plans—sales plans, supply chain plans, financial plans, etc. Of all our supply chain strategy engagements, we found this to be the biggest hurdle and very often needed a senior leadership mandate to align processes and plans. When we were successful in bringing them into one room for a meeting, the combined team created wonders. I have seen a stakeholder's excitement at the very first meeting after hearing familiar challenges being discussed by another colleague and how they successfully overcame it. They all found the integrated plan much more useful, even when eliminating some of the risks or constraints in the siloed plan. This Integrated Business Planning (IBP) is a cross-functional planning process for the entire organization.

The IBP is a process which involves all key aspects of demand, supply and financial analysis in the mid-to-long-term planning and decision-making process. This makes it uniquely cross-functional and multi-dimensional, and inherently better suited to help achieve the organization's business goals and strategy. IBP planning covers the medium-term planning horizon which is neither addressed by the annual operating planning process nor the long-term strategic plan—this is what makes it so unique. Different planning processes, their horizons and key components of the IBP process are shown in the diagram in Figure 4.14.

IBP translates the strategic plan and multiple functional plans into an actionable plan for the entire organization, which leads to a better execution. This is also a decision-making process which considers medium-term strategy, financial plans, scenario evaluation, portfolio management, demand and supply elements. The process is characterized by a culture of trust, cross-functional collaboration and teamwork in a minimum time horizon of 18–24 months.

IBP not only sets up a process or plan, but establishes a thorough review mechanism to ensure a value creation (see Figure 4.15).

The review process tracks strategic business decision parameters such as revenue trend, market share and profits trends, and customer happiness. It also tracks other key operational metrics such as inventory levels, short orders, overtime, inter-plant transfers, expediting, reduced order fulfillment, poor resource utilization, etc.

Implementation

Given the overarching nature of the IBP process, which cuts across multiple functions to establish a capability, it needs a robust implementation

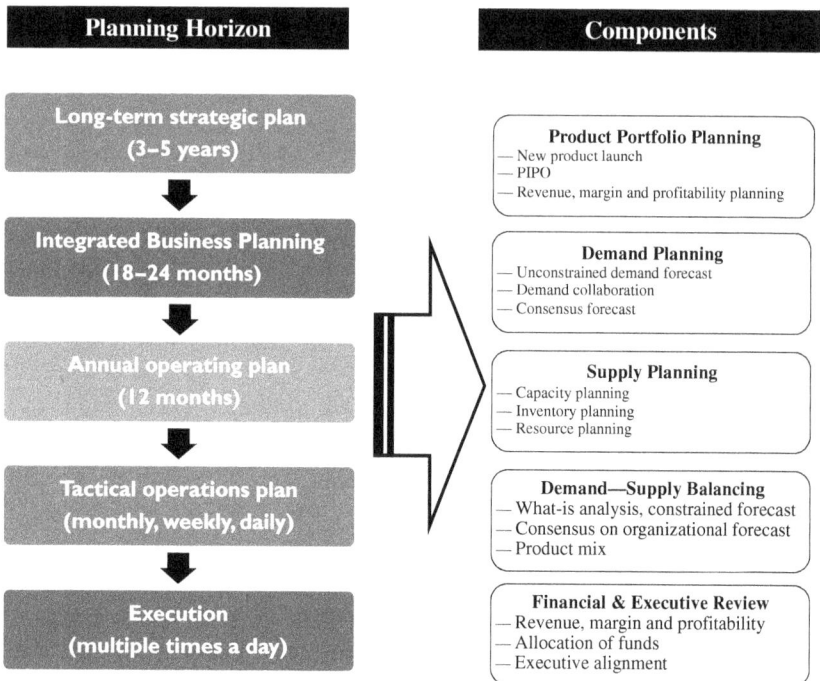

FIGURE 4.14   Integrated business planning elements.

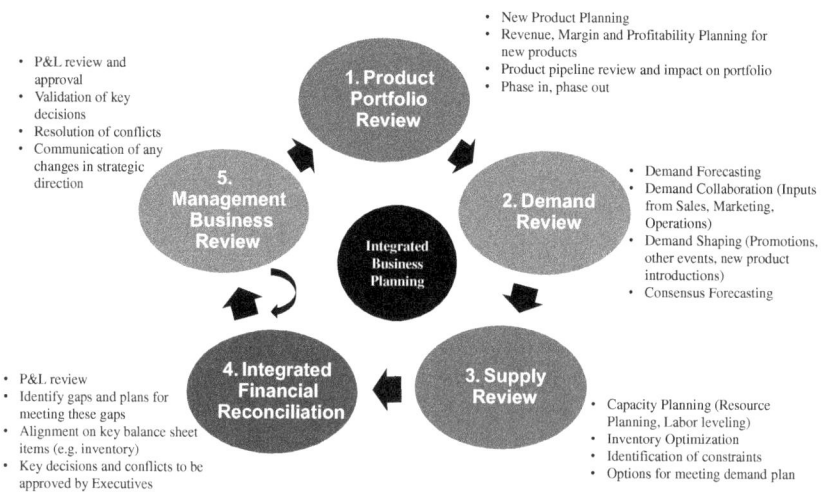

FIGURE 4.15   Integrated business planning process.

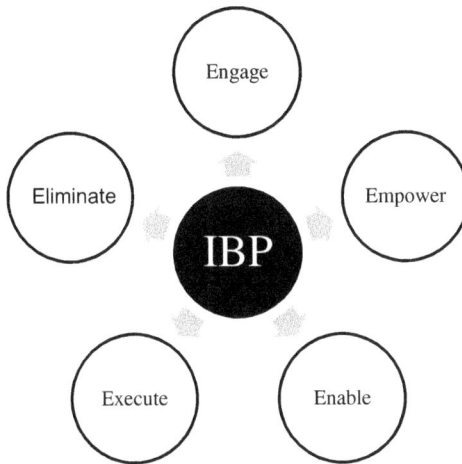

FIGURE 4.16 Integrated business planning implementation.

method. We have established a "5-E Approach" to implement IBP in an organization for faster realization of benefits (see Figure 4.16).

Engage

To ENGAGE is to identify the members of the core team and align them on the benefits of IBP (Integrated Business Plan). The ENGAGE phase involves the following activities:

- Define capabilities across the functional boundaries and quantify the targets for the IBP roll-out
- Involve the key stakeholders in the IBP process and give a baseline for the IBP roll-out schedule
- Set clear expectations, job definitions, organization design, and process ownerships and define a communication plan for all the stakeholders
- Align all the functions to the common goal instead of working for own bonus aspirations. Sales and marketing typically provide conservative forecasts; the supply chain function may inflate forecasts to justify longer production runs and greater factory efficiencies.

It is therefore critical to evaluate and then identify the right set of people to "engage", so that they can break free from their functional silos and drive, not only themselves, but also others towards the common goals of the organization.

Empower

To EMPOWER is to provide the selected people with the authority to make key decisions and resolve conflict, while driving the imminent changes.

- Clear definition of roles and responsibilities—there is often a lack of alignment on who takes the call on the final forecast and who resolves conflicts across multiple functions
- Reward and consequences—there can be misaligned incentives across different functions. The core team should be empowered to change the incentives if this is required. For example, a sales representative is incentivized on the sales volume; a supply chain person is incentivized on the lowered cost of execution. A conflict arises if an organization receives an emergency order and the shipment needs to be expedited as that impacts one of their goals negatively.
- Skills and tools—empowerment is needed to define new working principles for better adoption of IBP
- Work flow and chain of authority specific to IBP—this must be visible and acceptable to all participants.

It is very important that the key participants in IBP are positioned as the leaders of the change and aligned to the requirements of the role. The Figure 4.16 shows that lack of alignment on any one of these capabilities can result in potential issues and even a poor adoption of the entire process.

Enable

To ENABLE is to make available the right tools, sharing the data, technology and analytics capabilities to drive IBP implementation. The technology aspect of IBP focuses on addressing this situation by enabling the "right" access to the "right" data by the "right" set of people.

The role of technology and analytics in enabling IBP can be summarized as follows:

- Multiple data sources within disparate systems is complex in nature, and Data Management and integration capabilities are required to ensure timely, complete and accurate data
- Multi-dimensional goals and views need to be aligned with different organizations within the company and aggregated and supported by IBP
- Technology can be leveraged to model, manage and monitor the multi-dimensional decision parameters with different levels of aggregation

- Modeling and simulation
- Building the financial models from volume-based models
- Profitability analysis for different channels, products and customers
- Extracting and consolidating data from underlying systems without the need for manual intervention
- Reporting and dissemination of results across different time dimensions, to allow daily monitoring and other timely decisions related to execution.

Execute

To EXECUTE is to implement IBP process steps and ensure that the group is continuously aligned on the benefits being accrued during the process. The importance of the EXECUTE part of the approach during the IBP implementation process cannot be overstated. Due to the amount of commitment required and the amount of change involved, it is not uncommon to feel frustrated with the process, especially when the benefits take some time to start accruing. It is not to be forgotten that the best tools and technology will not have the desired impact unless the execution of the IBP process is flawless.

Often the perception is that IBP is a "supply chain" process, which could not be farther from the truth. IBP enablement requires not only a strong executive sponsorship but also leadership involvement for its success. From a process perspective, several new capabilities have to be developed such as:

- Aligning on a planning calendar. Clear visibility is needed of when a certain set of information is needed or when a certain meeting is happening. Often the most successful companies will have a defined and published calendar for at least the next two quarters
- Visibility beyond the end of the fiscal year. As the planning horizon for IBP meetings is often 18–24 months, organizations need to develop capabilities in underlying planning processes such as Demand Planning, Supply Planning, Financial Planning, Account Planning, Trade Promotion Planning, etc. to cover this planning horizon
- Clearly aligned roles, responsibilities and inputs for key information reviewed during each of these meetings
- A structured process to prepare for each of the meetings. Since each of the meetings is designed to achieve certain business objectives and is very limited in duration, it is critical to focus discussion on decision points, critical assumptions and where there are chances of likely exceptions in the process.

Eliminate

This step sounds a bit drastic but given the pharmaceutical business situation, we recommend a process step in the method in order to make some hard calls. As the supply chain directly impacts on the company's topline and bottom-line growth, the tolerance limit is very short. The IBP process quickly understands the success or failure of people, process or tools and helps to make training or rotation plans. This step ensures that an organization has well-defined performance measurement criteria for faster decision-making such as:

• People performance scorecard
• Process effectiveness scorecard
• System evaluations and audits.

Adoption and implementation of IBP is often a journey instead of a "big-bang" implementation. As described in previous sections, multiple capabilities are required for successful implementation and all may not come in a single go. This process also has a medium-term goal which at times creates frustration for many stakeholders as they do not see immediate benefits. We recommend that an initial assessment is done to find out how mature the planning processes are and where the major gaps are in capabilities across people, process and technology. This also helps in creating the benchmark on which the IBP success or failure would be measured.

We have learned several lessons through the IBP implementations—here are a few of them:

• Get executive alignment and sponsorship early
• Identify a process champion that will lead the overall IBP process
• The process around volume forecast needs to be improved first. Therefore steps such as product portfolio review, demand review and supply review should be addressed before others
• Agreement is needed on the planning horizon across all functional areas. Although IBP requires a planning horizon of 18–24 months, organizations are often not in a position to perform volume, cost and revenue forecasting for such a long planning horizon because of existing limitations across several areas. Often organizations start with a 9–12 months horizon and then slowly extend the planning horizon
• Integration of the financial forecasting process with the volume forecasting process is needed. Once the volume forecasting capabilities have been developed, integration with the financial planning process needs to be established so that decisions can be taken on the basis of financial metrics such as margins, operating profit, cash flow, etc.

The industry is moving from larger to smaller organizations as indicated by several recent spin-offs. Product strategy is shifting from the blockbuster drugs to smaller revenue-based drugs—many orphan drugs' approval in the recent past proves that. Healthcare reports in many countries across the world show that the focus is moving from product to patient. All these changes will have a significant impact on the pharmaceutical supply chain system. The supply chain of the future will be built around efficiency, flexibility, responsiveness and predictive capabilities that will fundamentally shift the supply chain paradigm from a cost optimization model to a value optimization model—the 5-5-5 Model: Connected Supply Chain would make this happen.

This part of the chapter was authored in collaboration with Sandeep Kumar. Sandeep is a supply chain strategist and has helped many clients across the globe to remodel their supply chains. He works with Infosys Limited.

IN DIGITAL WE TRUST: INDUSTRIALIZE CUSTOMER CENTRICITY

The day starts a bit wired for Tina—low grade fever, a light-headed feeling and nausea. She doesn't feel good at all and sits in her room in a New York City hotel, feeling very depressed. It's a Tuesday, an extremely busy work day for her—she can't afford to wait to find out what's wrong with her; she needs to get better as soon as possible—there's a lot to finish before she can head home on the Thursday evening flight. Tina opens her laptop, googles her symptoms to get hundreds of matching conditions within seconds. She gets a fairly good idea about what it could be by visiting Wikipedia, a few medical websites, a couple of product sites and several patients' and physicians' blogs. Her smart brain starts processing the warm sensibilities from the world of the internet and she is already starting to feel better. She finds she has enough courage to get up and make a cappuccino, her favorite and available in the hotel room. Her brain starts working better—she needs to see a doctor just to be sure that it's nothing serious. Now, how to find a physician in this strange city who will be willing to see her at just a few hours' notice? She desperately looks for a physician online using her iPhone social networking apps, but it's bad news—she can't find anyone nearby.

There is another side to it. My wife doesn't allow me to check the internet when I feel sick. And for good reason—the conclusion is invariably that I very well could be terminally ill, and should be rushed to the nearest emergency treatment center. Of course, it's not entirely the internet's fault. I suppose I might tend to assume the worst, or at least consider what the worst case scenario could be.

I don't think I'm alone. I've often heard people joke that, whatever their symptoms, medical sites will tell them they probably have a terrible illness. But the reality is that we are only at the frontier of the convergence of medicine and the web, and things are improving very, very quickly.

There are close to two billion people like Tina looking for information on the internet. Of these, about 80% are in social network sites in the US. Unfortunately, only 10% of physicians are on social network sites ...mostly for clinical work. At the moment, regulatory boundaries do vary from country to country and don't allow a stronger connection to be made between patient, physician and pharmaceutical manufacturer, but it won't be long before this can happen—the digital world will change it all.

Highly educated patients will play a significant role in future decision-making. They will research all aspects of a disease, as well as the treatment options, product options and price benefits before they see a physician. They will also look at online chat with physicians before spending a lot of time and money visiting a doctor, going through the analysis and ending up paying out a huge amount of money to the inflated cost of healthcare.

The digital revolution has had an exponential impact on the opportunities for companies to deliver their brand messages in an increasingly wide variety of channels and variants, creating in its wake a torrent of data detailing their customers' interactions at every stage. The speed and relative low cost of creating and delivering marketing messages through digital channels, as opposed to traditional media like television, print and direct mail, has enabled companies to build a vast digital property whose growth and development have often outpaced their ability to govern it and harness the data created by it in a manner that allows them to truly leverage its capabilities. When this accelerated growth is applied to an enterprise selling a multitude of brands across the globe, each with its own unique set of ever-growing digital property and evolving audience segments, and all delivering their messages through a multitude of tools operated by even more advertising agencies, it is no surprise that the result is often an enormous decrease in potential efficiency, high levels of redundancy of effort and higher regulatory risks. This has led to a new way of thinking in the world of digital operations—that of the factory manager who is able to manage huge numbers of production lines from raw material through to final delivery to the customer on a global scale, continuously increasing efficiency and quality at every step. This approach has allowed many pharmaceutical companies to take back control of their "digital production line" and to start finally realizing the promised benefits of the digital revolution, enabling multi-channel marketing, the promises of increased accuracy of message targeting, increased speed to market and better understanding of their customers. And everything delivered with 100% compliance and at decreased delivery cost.

How Did We Get Here?

Not so very long ago, we marketers led much simpler, more relaxed lives. We had our brands and a nice set of segments where everyone in the world fitted neatly into one or the other, and a fairly limited number of channels to get our marketing messages across to our segments. Media plans that detailed all the newspapers, magazines and television shows we would advertise in were created for an entire year in advance. All this was terribly expensive and, by today's standards, slow paced. To make matters worse, we couldn't ever really know for certain what the effect of our work was. Of course, we could measure the general "lift" in sales following an advertising campaign, but we couldn't be sure which mix of channels and messages were exactly right to get the best results—we could only take an educated guess. This wasn't that bad if you weren't very good at marketing. Since the links between marketing activity and sales were spotty at best, it was easier for the "not very good" marketers to make sure that they were never to blame for a sales slump, and that they were certainly accountable for any increases in sales. Then some damned fool went and invented the internet and the game got very complex and very hard.

The growth of the internet in terms of global adoption has been staggering. Relatively cheap public access, particularly with the dominance of internet-enabled mobile phones penetrating even the poorest countries, combined with low barriers to entry for online business, has fueled exponential growth in usage and the creation of digital content. The acceleration is so rapid that writing down statistics for a publication such as this one is a bit like an astronaut sending a postcard with their current speed only a second after lift-off … by the time anyone reads it, it will be old news. Yet we are still only at the very beginning of the digital age. Less than half the world is online at all, never mind being addicted to Facebook, Twitter, Pinterest and the rest. As adoption continues to spread across the globe, the digital landscape we must navigate as marketers will not only become increasingly complex, but it is likely that the very nature of the medium itself will change as new cultures embrace these new modes of communication and develop their own online tools, platforms, networks and devices to add to the vast production already being generated.

At the early stages of this digital evolution, when people were starting to realize the potential the internet could play in the world of marketing and advertising, there were some promises made. They were all about efficiency. The people selling online advertising showed us how we could set up campaigns for pennies on the dollar, set an exact number of people who would see our advertisements, and specify very accurately where our ads would appear. It was just like placing a high-end travel ad aimed at ABC1s in the National Geographic, but it could be done for USD 500 instead of USD 5000, it could all be set up in a few days instead of requiring advanced booking six months out, and the internet people would "guarantee" the number of people who would see our ads (or at least who would see the page where our ad was placed). And now, even more excitingly, we could actually know how many people clicked on our ad! This was all very fulfilling when we could announce in a meeting that a certain percentage had clicked on our ad, so they must be very interested in our brand, and if they all bought something from us, we must have made thousands and thousands of dollars, all for an investment of just USD 500. Surely we must spend more!

Digital advertising continued to become more advanced, allowing marketers to select different messages to show different audiences, at first based on geography and eventually based on what they ordered for their breakfast. Analytics went from expensive, sophisticated tools that marketers couldn't understand to simple, free tools that anyone can use and understand. However, further adoption of multi-channel marketing adds more complexity to data and information needs.

All of this super-fast growth should be good news if you are in marketing and your mission is to tell the story of your brand, or brands, to as many people in your target markets as often and as cheaply as possible. And for many, it really was a huge advance in the way we connect with our customers. But the rapid adoption and permutation of everything digital across everything we do resulted in just as much confusion and complication as it did in efficiency.

The number of tools developed to help marketers achieve various tasks online continues to increase. New tools become outdated within a year of deployment. And, although a business might benefit from all the future upgrades a tool or product offers to ensure it stays relevant, other tools are constantly coming along that are better, do more, or work better when integrated with other tools. It's a bit like choosing a mobile phone. You pick the one you think is best, based not only on the phone as you see it in the store, but based on all the apps that work well with it and how often you think it will be upgraded with new features, etc. Enterprise marketing tools are no different in principle. But in most businesses, especially the large Fortune 500s we tend to deal with in the consulting trade, marketing tools in place can easily be up to 50 different products, all designed to do very specific things. Some work well together and do just fine "out of the box". Some require expensive integrations and/or customization work to behave the way we want them to behave. All this creates an extremely complex digital ecosystem, and we've only talked about technology so far, never mind the people and processes needed to actually make it all work.

A Common Set of Problems

Since we are discussing the concept of industrializing digital delivery in this chapter, let's put the above description of the enterprise with 50 marketing tools all in place, at various states of integration and customization, into context. What we have is a very large factory with an array of machines that all do one general thing, which is "digital marketing." But so far in our story, there are no people in the factory, so the machines don't do anything useful, as they all either a) need to be continually told what to do, b) need to at least first be programmed to do things based on some set of rules or information from another machine, or c) capture data that is intended for people to read, understand, and put to use. So let's make it a bit more complex and add some humans!

The people in these large enterprise systems come from a huge variety of backgrounds, technology product companies and geographies. The people come from disciplines like digital marketing, brand management, CRM, eCommerce, system architecture, development, and quality assurance groups. These disciplines also come with all manner of variety, sub-disciplines and at different maturity levels. The entire group will normally be made of some mixture of the company's own staff, advertising agencies, systems integrators, and consultancies. And to make it even more complex, they will be spread out all around the world.

In most cases, there are many groups of people, usually ad agencies, who all do very similar tasks, only in different parts of the world, or for different business units or brands within the company. However, the way all these tasks are done and just how well they are done can vary wildly, as well as the tools that are used. So, now we have a huge factory full of machines, and a much larger number of people who all want to use the machines in different ways and at different times. But the real dilemma is this: the people are all divided into little groups who rarely talk to one another—especially those who actually operate the machines. And the people in charge of the production lines—both specifying what is produced and managing volume and delivery to customers—are also in separate groups that rarely talk.

This brings us finally to the processes within our factory. Remember that one of the big promises of the internet to us as marketers was a huge increase in efficiency. And anyone who has studied the manufacturing industry knows very well how important process and efficiency are in a factory. This is probably one of the single most important, and most frequently missing, aspects of the huge enterprise digital ecosystems I have come across—the lack of clear and measured processes that ensure that everything that moves through the factory does so as efficiently as possible and at the highest level of quality. There may be processes to produce single products, like a single marketing campaign in one country for one brand, but when the people in charge start using all the machines for many different purposes, and running many localized variants of several campaigns simultaneously, the processes for efficiency just aren't there.

The final result of this all-too-common scenario is pretty much the opposite of what we marketers were expecting from the digital revolution. Yes, the tools we now have can do amazing things and, if used properly, can certainly result in greater efficiency. But the reality is often a rapidly rising cost to maintain and improve our digital ecosystems, and loss of control over how our marketing messages are created, delivered and measured.

The Quality of Digital Marketing

So far, we have talked a lot about efficiency, which is probably not the first thing that most people in the marketing profession are known to focus on. But that is only because of the context we are using of a "factory" model for marketing operations. Really, we are talking about Reach, Audience Segmentation, and Relevance. And specifically, how we maximize delivery of messages to our audience, create a deep understanding of what our customers want, and then tailor and deliver messaging and content that engages them in such a way as to make them loyal advocates of our brand or brands—the entire area of customer centricity. All as efficiently as possible—and in today's market that means super-fast delivery to market at the lowest possible cost, all while maintaining quality. The frequency in which these are done is equally important to make the model successful.

Now, most engineers will tell you that you can have it done quickly, or you can have it done well—pick one. So any model that is therefore designed to produce something very fast and very cheap, and not only good but *better*, is going to have to work very hard indeed! As modern six-sigma thinking challenges the use of "and" instead of "or", the factory model benefits from the resulting speed, lower cost and quality.

Quality means many different things in this context, and it is highly critical. In a broad sense, quality coming out of a digital marketing operations factory often refers to:

1. Branding—have all the brand style guidelines been followed carefully, through each channel and in each variation around the world?
2. Timing—are global campaigns well-orchestrated? Can the operation deliver messaging both quickly and in synch with offline campaign activity on both a global and local level?
3. Localization—can the operation deliver on branding and timing, as well as shaping and translating campaign messaging for localized audiences and deliver through local as well as global channels?
4. Targeting and Testing—are messages and content customized-based on audience behaviour? Can the operation test variations across campaigns, countries and segments to continuously improve the brands' ability to engage their audience members in a meaningful and personalized way?
5. Analytics and Insight—with all the hundreds of moving parts and interactions in this ecosystem, can the operation effectively use web analytics to deliver clear, succinct and actionable insights that help brand managers improve their marketing?

All these capabilities help enable a multi-channel marketing capability for a company. Fully integrated channels and effective interactions between the company and customers through multiple channels can improve the brand revenue significantly. I describe this integrated and interactive multi-channel marketing as "i2 MCM". In fact, I think most people would agree that it is much better to produce one outstanding campaign than 50 average ones. After all, we are competing for people's attention amongst an increasingly vast background of messages, both digital and traditional, each vying for our audience's attention.

Industrial-Strength Solutions

The ability to drive both efficiency and quality through an enormous digital ecosystem was a clear need for global enterprises everywhere.

And there are many ways different companies have approached the problem with varying success. However, it was the pharmaceutical industry that made some very significant gains early in this arena, and now has some concrete examples of true "digital industrialization" that are able to deliver on many of the promises of the digital age.

The models that are working well in the pharmaceutical industry are powerful, well-organized end to end services that can be delivered in factory style operations that blend people, process and technology. On the technology front, digital platforms are forming the central hub that manages all the company's digital property, delivers messages, and processes data. On the people and process side, organizations are decoupling traditional digital marketing activities based on skills required to assign each task to the most efficient operator while building global delivery capabilities that are driving speed to market at reduced cost.

The Digital Industry Within Your Company

You need to create a digital industry within your organization to create differentiated values. Like any other industry, this will have its Production operation, Marketing, Demand creators, Quality Management, Governance, R&D and Management functions.

Leadership/Management ensures a digital vision for the company (see Figure 4.17). Send leadership communications to set the expectation of managing all digital and mobile work through this operation. This makes it easy to create the demand for digital operations without conflicting with any existing execution set-up.

The Governance & PMO team ensures leadership vision is being executed in the operations. This function is more hands-on to ensure change management, risk and issues management, and regulatory compliance and select and evaluate delivery partners through a partner accreditation program. They are also responsible for managing financials in the operation and ensure financial value creation by meeting a cost savings target.

The model most common in large pharmaceutical digital ecosystems today combines a robust and scalable global delivery hub with decoupled marketing tasks. This requires excellence in the formation of partnerships on the part of all parties involved, as the model invariably has vendors all around the world collaborating with the enterprise. In extreme cases, we have seen over 50 advertising agencies spread worldwide all working through a single delivery hub. As with any well-run factory, there is a very well-articulated design for Governance, Roles and Responsibilities, KPIs and SLAs for the factory's performance, standard

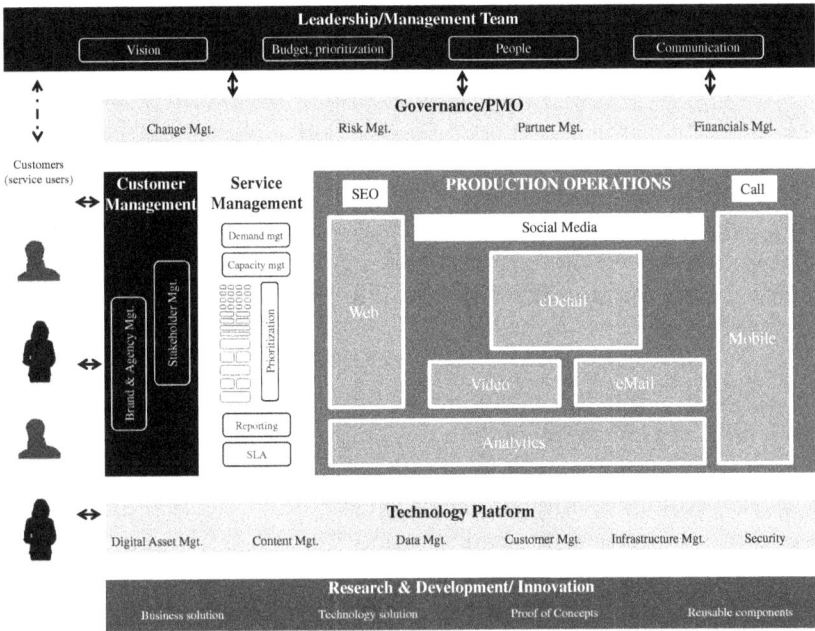

FIGURE 4.17

operating procedures, quality assurance, demand planning, and continuous improvement of quality and efficiency.

Since these operations centralize digital activity, there is also a significant amount of thought and effort put into "onboarding" of partners. This is typical of new ad agencies who will be working with the hub to deliver digital work, and need to understand how to work with the group.

Operating Team

Experience tells me that a digital operation should be built in such a way that it can work seamlessly at low work volume and scale when work volume increases or needs expansion into multiple geographies. This needs the right governance and operating model which is flexible enough to accommodate demand variances.

It is a good idea to have leaders for all key service areas in the operation. The leaders can either be from the pharmaceutical company internal or a combination of internal and outsourced partner organizations if work is delivered by partners. In the beginning we recommend an overall operations leader as the captain of the ship. This person can wear several hats in the beginning if volume is low including PMO, service management and client management. But as the operation grows it needs several people as program leader, client manager, demand manager, agency and brand manager and PMO leader. This model recommends having an overall production operations manager with several leads working within this role. These roles are as managers for various production units, e.g. Web, Mobile, Social, eMail or eDetail. Test leads, data management leads, release managers and regulatory submission managers are also part of this team. The bandwidth requirement entirely depends on the demand.

I strongly recommend having a dedicated Quality & Compliance (Q&C) team. This team defines processes, SOP, checklists and guidelines and ensures operations are fully compliant with external and internal regulatory requirements at the country level. The data privacy and information security is a key challenge in the digital and mobile world which needs to be handled carefully. This Q&C team monitors service level agreements to drive productivity improvements. This role also carries out compliance audits to keep the operations work compliant at all times.

There should be an innovation lead to drive innovation in the digital world. Digital and mobile technologies are so fast-changing that dedicated effort is needed to keep the operations up to date with the latest happenings. This team keeps operations innovative by connecting with other organizations, tracking industry and newer technology availability to eliminate obsolescence.

Operating Model

The global nature of the pharmaceutical operation demands that the digital operations support marketing projects around the world. A hub and spoke model creates the ability to service all markets and provides time zone-friendly support around the world.

In the beginning, this model can even operate in a specific therapeutic area in one country and can then expand to accommodate various brands in multiple geographies. It can easily be customized for a company affiliate and adapted into multi-channel delivery channels. While this model is flexible, I recommend a crawl-walk-run approach to expand for better adoption.

The hub should be created for a business function or an affiliate, or in a geography where work volume is high. The major production hub can be created at an offshore location such as India which

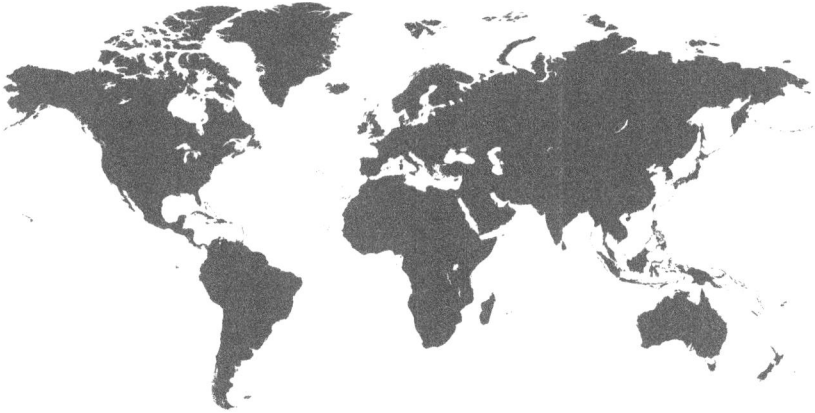

FIGURE 4.18   Hub and spoke delivery model.

supports all regional hubs in a "follow the sun" production model. A small production team can be onsite in the country hubs for the customer management, agency liaison, demand management, requirement gathering and carrying out of technical work on a smaller scale. As the operation model matures, the production staff levels in high cost locations will be reduced. The offshore hub can provide the flex capacity to support demand spikes across other hubs. Customer-facing roles such as project managers and service leads can be staffed in the spoke locations connected to a hub (see Figure 4.18). These teams will be supported by the hubs for project execution, training/accreditation, and support issue resolution and specialty service requests. The exact staffing needs and ramp-up plan can be determined based on the project demand. The spoke countries may have onsite production capability during specific periods in a year (POA, etc.) to meet seasonal digital demand. The digital marketing technologists need to be embedded within the brand teams who work very closely with the "factory" operation.

Crawl-Walk-Run Phases

The operating model with the right people, process, tools and established governance in a region should be matured before expanding into all business units or geographies. As every company and even every business function in an organization has its own way of managing marketing operations, the adoption cycle varies significantly. The recommendation is not to rush the expansion process, but not to go too slowly either which cuts momentum significantly.

	Setup Phase 8–10 weeks	Phase 1: 8–24 weeks	Phase 2: 25–60 weeks	Phase 3: >60 weeks
Strategic focus	Ops service design, communication and initial demand creation	Scale-up the Ops for few brands in multiple channels in a large market, e.g. US (taking US as an example for this model)	Scale-up the Ops to all brands in multiple channels in the US/ onboard few global brands	Global operations using best in class process, tools and people to ensure asset reuse, improve quality and reduce cost
Process & governance	• Ops service menu • SOP, checklist, guidelines • Brand & Agency communication • Technology strategy • Governance structure, roles & responsibilities • KPI, reporting	• Establish a steady project demand • Create Agency change management • Plan improvement initiatives • Finalize SLA and reporting • Establish compliance & quality mgt structure • Establish a pricing/ chargeback model	• Steady state PMO/steering operations • Finalize pricing/ chargeback • Full QM, compliance, security services • Establish FDA/HA package creation • Start productivity tracking	• Long-term Ops envisioning • Steady state PMO/steering • Measure operational improvement • Ensure "100% compliant" operation • Optimize operating model, pricing, SLA, and more
Service activation & adoption	• Activate subset of services to specific projects (Crawl) • Identify brands and agencies to work as a startup/ pilot • Communicate brands • Create demand plan for wave 1	• Activate end-to-end services to larger set of projects (Walk) • Communicate Agencies and conduct training sessions • Define ramp-up/down models • Carry out existing SOW assessment for cost saving opportunities • Create adoption planning—Agency accreditation program	• Execute all US (example) projects (Run) • Identify international projects • Communicate/ train all agencies including international locations • Define models to meet local needs • Activate change management at the country level	• Constantly focus on global relationship • Improve demand management • Onboard new brand/ agencies
Execution and Improvement	• Identify early adopter projects • Understand requirements of early adopter projects • Create estimation, staffing details • Set up tools/systems for early projects; Establish a support model	• Execute projects in shared services • Establish model-driven delivery mechanism—development, test, metadata, validation, release • Start asset reuse • Transition existing apps	• Development, support and maintenance of all marketing assets & applications • Establish production using integrated technology platform • Establish high reuse of assets	• Optimize Global delivery model • Establish franchise models
Innovation & maturity	• Define business & technology innovation structure • Establish technology architecture/ digital/mobile device strategy	• Identify tools/systems to improve mobile Factory operations—DAM/workflow/ Analytics, etc	• Establish integrated digital/mobile platform • Establish best in class technology adoption • Pilot solutions to increase business value	• Offer better solutions through newer technologies • Constantly keep Ops upgraded with the latest needs

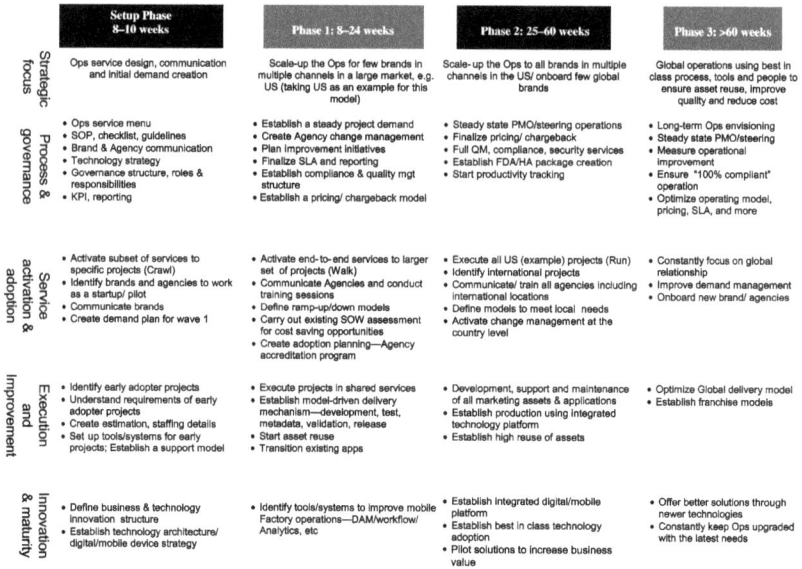

FIGURE 4.19 Crawl-Walk-Run roadmap.

Don't be super-rigid on operating processes—they may need tweaks to fit into different business units/affiliates/geographies based on their adoption pattern. As an example, for a brand with a highly matured brand–agency relationship, the operations can only offer technology services—testing and metadata management—to start engaging with the brand and build a relationship. The factory will go with full-service operation once the working relationship has been established. The other way of testing a new expansion is to run smaller pilots from an existing hub. This helps in fine-tuning operational parameters for the new business area to achieve higher customer satisfaction.

The chart in Figure 4.19 depicts an example of a crawl-walk-run plan.

Digital Platforms

The term "digital platform" is being used widely these days, and there is no precise definition that clearly states exactly what constitutes one. Generally speaking, a digital platform is an integrated system, typically heavily customized for a business's specific needs, which controls digital content, messaging and the resulting data. Content Management Systems (CMS), Digital Asset Management (DAM) systems, Marketing Automation tools, Customer Relationship Management (eCRM) systems, Campaign/Project Management tools and Analytics tools typically form the root of a relatively mature platform. The i2MCM (integrated and interactive multi-channel marketing) can integrate social media-driven customer data with the SFA data. The essence of these platforms is to allow global enterprises to use technology to deliver highly personalized, targeted, and engaging user experiences for their customers while continually building market intelligence that increases the effectiveness of those experiences.

The more sophisticated platforms found at leading pharmaceutical companies extend into social networks and integrate with them. These integrations often include: the ability to "listen" for conversations about a brand across hundreds of networks and then allow marketers to actively participate in them; the ability to share and publish content fluidly between owned digital property and social networks to create integrated campaigns and experiences; and the creation of a link and data trail between customers' activity on the company's sites and other networks. These integrations allow a form of "social CRM", where companies can learn much more about customer behavior and how to best engage with them.

This understanding of customer behavior is one of the factors that have moved leading companies ahead of the curve. Since these digital platforms connect to all digital marketing activity, from social integration to email campaigns to the hundreds of sites, microsites, and landing pages, to all manner of display advertising and everything in between, the data produced is mind-boggling. Indeed, it is the production of these huge sets of data and such a large array of tools, users and sites producing them that led so many companies to a state of complete confusion and near-paralysis when it came to data-based decision-making: there was just too much data for anyone to effectively use. This is where the analytics capabilities of the truly game-changing platforms come in.

The leading digital platforms are now able to create streamlined customer information—a single view of the customer that aggregates all customer behavioral data across all digital systems and presents it in a meaningful and useful manner to brand marketers. This data is extremely useful, as it gives a brand team the insights that digital has always promised, but without the headache and cost of extensive data analysis that is, to this day, the norm for many large enterprises grappling with "big data". When constructing the systems that provide unified customer views, marketers specify the metrics that are important to them—those that are supported with a business case showing how a marketer could use a metric to improve their marketing efforts—along the customer journey from basic brand awareness through loyalty and advocacy. The team building the digital platform then identifies each system and tool that will be generating customer data, and these days almost every piece of marketing software you can buy comes with some reporting or analytics feature, and integrates it into a single, multi-dimensional data warehouse that can build a complete picture of each customer's interactions and behaviors throughout the enterprise's ecosystem.

More customer knowledge creates some very powerful opportunities for the marketing team to engage with customers and deliver the highly personalized experiences at the efficiency rates that have been completely out of reach until recently. The brand team's interface into the digital platform considers a traditional marketing funnel where marketers try to move consumers from Awareness to Interest to Engaged to Transacting to Loyalty and then to Advocacy, and then overlays critical data into each phase that indicates what actions the marketer should take. Many platforms even offer detailed guidelines right inside the user interface (for the marketer) that describe what certain metrics might indicate and what specific strategies should be employed in the circumstance. This single view across all digital channels also gives marketers a better understanding of their segments and how their behavior changes by channel. For example, since they are able to measure responsiveness and engagement levels across segments and channels, they can now construct much more accurate Media Mix Analysis (MMA) models for digital. This ability to understand the effect of shifting investment in various digital media and its result at a very granular level then enables predictive analysis to a very high degree of accuracy, essentially helping marketers make budget and resource decisions that are both based on solid historical data and are predicted to have a strong ROI with confidence. Previously, MMA and predictive analytics was often an inexact science in most marketing departments, and the job of getting meaningful and useful statistics was painful, long and expensive. Now, although the use of these platforms for MMA and predictive analysis is still only emerging in maturity, we have taken great strides in our ability to finally realize some of the key benefits of digital marketing.

As well as helping marketers make smarter decisions and understand their customers better, the platform can also integrate the customer analytics with content targeting and marketing automation tools to create deeply personalized user experiences on a global scale. In the case of content, the platforms allow marketing teams to create business rules that will then govern what kind of content a user will see. The possibilities are nearly endless, but common approaches include:

- The placement of specific content we think the user might be interested in, based on some previous action. This includes up-selling and cross-selling rules based on products a user has searched for and/or viewed, as well as promotion of that product to the user later in their session, or even for the next time they return to the site, if they didn't buy

- Serving different content, or varying styles of content, based on the user's segment (given that they are either recognized or logged in) based on what has historically had the best result.

In the case of marketing automation, particularly in the field of lead generation and nurturing, the streamlined customer data is also extremely powerful. These automation tools are becoming more and more prevalent in nearly all industries, and are being used widely in the pharmaceutical sector where they can satisfy the hybrid marketing needs of B2C (Business to Consumer) of over the counter drugs and the more usual B2B (Business to Business) for prescription drugs business models. In a B2B model, these systems are best set up to create a single, integrated Sales and Marketing funnel, where leads generated from digital marketing activity are passed into a sales CRM system where they are scored to determine whether they are "sales ready" (a sales rep should call on them) or should be placed in the nurturing system, where automated marketing messages will be delivered to them, based on a set of business rules that is designed to engage the prospect to the point where they do become "sales ready". This saves considerable time and effort for the sales force, allowing them to focus on prospects ready to buy while never letting potential new customers fall through the cracks. In B2C models, the lead nurturing systems are a pure digital marketing tool, sending customized messaging—typically email and targeted onsite content—to customers based on some set of rules.

In both the cases above, the ability to run A/B or more complex multivariate tests should always be considered a foundational element of a digital platform. Large enterprises have a significant advantage here, in that their vast digital property allows them to run tests that become statistically significant very quickly, due to the high volume of users and digital property being tested. Tests are run continuously, across channels and segments, to deliver deeper and deeper insight into the effectiveness of every aspect of digital content and delivery. It is often the results of these tests that will help shape the business rules marketing teams use to target content and govern marketing automation tools. The insights from testing will tell marketers how best to engage with each segment, not only in general, but in each channel, or in each country or even based on what stage of the marketing funnel they are in. This brings our ability to understand our customers to a level which previously only very small businesses could achieve, but on a global scale. Whereas before we might only have understood what kind of messaging and channels would work best for some generic segment, like "ABC1s", now we can understand the difference between what marketing is effective when targeting past customer ABC1s in France, shopping on our mobile app, vs. ABC1s in Germany, who are shopping on Google and aren't even aware of our product. You can easily see the breadth of variation possible—and it could become extremely complex. But dealing with this kind of complexity, and making it simple, is exactly what really good digital platforms do.

This platform, if we are to again consider the context of a "factory", encompasses the entire factory and all the machines inside it. The fundamental difference is that, rather than a whole series of separate assembly lines, there is something more like a single assembly line capable of producing a huge variation of content and messaging intelligently.

Why This Model Works?

This digital and mobile operation is designed for better value creation. This industrialized solution breaks down end to end work by skills, enabling the best people to do the work as per their skills as opposed to being forced to do everything in the operation that comes their way. This model brings in new capabilities to the digital operations world to make the solution complete. The operation also becomes the house of Capability Center of Excellences (CC) to constantly improve operations.

Decoupling—Skill-Based Work Rationalization

Integral to this model is the notion of decoupling marketing activity and specialization. Essentially, this breaks down the creation of campaigns, for example, into specific tasks, and then assigns each task to a team that is best suited to delivering it. In many cases, companies not using some form of decoupling are paying their ad agencies top rates to carry out work that can be done for a fraction of the cost and better by someone else. For example, while it makes sense to pay an agency high rates for creative concepts, branding, and visual design, it does not make sense to pay that same agency the same high rates to build digital property already specified, test it (in the software development QA and UAT sense), validate compliance for legal mandates, create multiple regionalized/translated variants, tag content, and deploy it. All those tasks are best done by technology delivery specialists, and can be done better, faster and cheaper using an offshore delivery model. On the other hand, disciplines and their related tools within the digital marketing realm are so varied that it pays to create centers of excellence that can focus on a single area—marketing automation using Eloqua for example—and become experts at using the tool to manage and deliver campaigns.

Specialism

If you start to examine the parts inside a global enterprise's digital ecosystem, you might find yourself feeling a little bit like the first quantum physicists must have felt. As you break down the ecosystem into smaller and smaller parts, each element contains more complexity, and moving parts, than you ever expected. The tools we have to use today are extremely complex, and almost always come with a huge set of additional features, plug-ins, endless upgrades, and so forth. Often, it seems like every company that once made, say, an email management tool is now trying to turn their tool into a proper marketing platform. Everything we buy comes with reports, enhanced targeting, automation capabilities, testing capabilities … and so on and so on. And, if we're feeling really sophisticated, we can start customizing the tools to do exactly what we want them to do, adding "rules engines" and feeding them data from other tools that tell them exactly when to send my friend Dave an invitation to my birthday.

The issue is that, given the complexity—and wonderful potential—of these tools, there is just no possible way we can master them and drive maximum value from them without creating Capability Centers of Excellence (CC). These CCs are very powerful, as they ensure that a company's investment in a tool is maximized for the life of the tool. There is a technical side, where the CC team can install the tool, manage integrations, manage upgrades, maintain and repair the tool, and take care of technical configurations and customizations. It is almost like having a master mechanic looking after your car—no matter how good the car is when you bring it home, there is no end of adjustments a good mechanic can make to make it run better, faster, and more comfortably.

The other side of the CC is related to mastery of campaign or content production and delivery. Now, what "production" means depends on the medium, but good digital factories can handle every channel. For example, the SEO CC will ensure all content that is created passes the strictest SEO criteria, from metadata to canonical tagging to target keyword density to structure within a site. An eCRMCC might manage an on-going cadence of segmented activation/re-activation rules, regionalized market pressure rules, and sales funnel optimization. The level of detail for any discipline can go very deep, and at a global scale, each additional layer of expertise adds up to further and further fine tuning of the digital operation, which translates directly into profit.

The operations running in the pharmaceutical industry today have a very successful mix of expert services at their core.

Just like other aspects of these factories, specialist CCs usually run a "core/flex" model, where there is a small core of subject matter experts and an extended, on-demand team that can quickly ramp up and ramp down to match fluctuating demand without carrying the large overhead costs of either hiring a large team of such experts or contracting a series of specialist agencies on an annual "agency of record" basis.

Common CCs and expert service suites include:

Web Optimization

Specialists in all aspects of user experience design, inbound marketing, and goal conversion strategy spend time analyzing site data to continuously enhance performance of digital property. This CC includes experts in SEO analysis and strategy, heuristic site analysis for user experience optimization factors (engagement, speed of goal attainment, abandonment causes, navigational and information architecture clarity and alignment with site purpose and goals), and goal path optimization through multivariate testing of content, messaging and visual design.

Portals, Landing Pages and Microsites

While these types of pages are typically conceived by creative design agencies, setting them up to be fully optimized both in terms of user engagement and goal conversion as well as taking into account data flow from systems like CRM and MDM, for personalization, analytics, and data integrity, are all critical tasks best left to Factory CCs. Indeed, these pages are often passed to the Web Optimization group mentioned above to then optimize them throughout the life of a campaign based on analytics evidence and A/B testing.

Mobile

Application development and building for the mobile web are disciplines that are gaining more and more traction, and require specialized design and development skills. Often, responsive design, although a good system, just isn't good enough when companies really want to optimize for the full range of mobile and tablet form factors. In cases like this, mobile UXD specialists often take up the production and variation side of a single design concept coming from a creative agency. This enables businesses to develop highly optimized mobile experiences without paying over the odds for a series of design variants for each device and browser.

In the pharmaceutical sector, mobile development is becoming one of the most sought-after services, especially for tablets. In many cases, entire field sales forces are swapping their old laptops for iPads, and with that comes the possibility of highly personalized, dynamic sales presentations. Digital factories excel in this arena, as they are able to take creative concepts and quickly turn them into winning sales tools in a matter of weeks, delivering them virtually to sales teams around the world, connecting data in the right way and enabling other CC skillsets to deliver closed-loop marketing solutions.

Online eDetailing

An extension of the Mobile sales tools is Online eDetailing, where doctors and other customers are able to review information on pharmaceuticals in their own time, using whichever device they prefer. Again, the factory approach ensures consistency of data and brand quality in all its rich varieties, tying information together across channels and building marketing intelligence inside the unified customer portal (UCP).

Metadata Tagging

Metadata and analytical data tagging and data management are core digital production factory offerings. All successful pharmaceutical factories establish a dedicated data and analytics team as part of the production line with specific, extensive pharmaceutical experience. We talked earlier about the vast data trails left behind by the explosion in digital property, and this is a key element to keeping it under control and being able to leverage the data created rather than becoming bound by it.

As anyone will tell you, "rubbish in, rubbish out". If data and content are not properly managed and tagged with a single taxonomy and approach, the amount of useful information the marketing team will be able to extract will diminish severely.

This is also relevant to digital asset management (DAM). Any DAM system should be viewed as a library, and any good library needs good librarians. This team in the factory production line acts as librarians, making sure everything is in order so that any system or person can find exactly what they are looking for—be it a piece of data that tells us how popular some content is or a tag that lets a creative agency find the perfect photo for a new landing page—and spare the cost of buying it or, more expensively, having a new photo shoot.

eCRM

eCRMCCs are an emerging concept in the pharmaceutical sector, although they are used extensively in Consumer packaged goods (CPG) and retail enterprise factories. Although the natural inclination is to leverage eCRM tools and capabilities in the OTC side of the pharmaceutical house, the more powerful option lies in social CRM and its use as a sales enabler. Teams inside these CCs will control marketing automation tools like Eloqua and Marketo, setting market pressure rules, re-activation rules, event-based marketing triggers, and so forth, based on a combination of strategy, analytics and a solid understanding of regional segment behavior. But, when we consider the symptom-based buying behavior of most customers who are purchasing OTC pharmaceuticals, it is clear that such eCRM tactics are never going to be as effective as when applied to the CPG and retail world. When we consider social CRM, however, and its use in building a map of sales target networks and enabling sales and marketing teams to gain deeper understanding of prescription drug customers, create meaningful interactions in discussions and forums, and then embed this intelligence in their sales CRM system, we have a winner. This is complex work, and turning data from the universe of social networks into actionable insights, attributes that prescribe or embellish segments or signify buying behavior is not for the faint-hearted. But when done correctly, as only a CC that is dedicated to this science can, there is a direct impact on the sales of prescription drugs, both as a result of sales representative understanding of their customer base and from the ability of the sales and marketing funnel to identify prospects' stages in the purchase path and appropriate actions (i.e. Nurture a Lead, Sales Ready, Re-Activate, etc.).

Value Creation Through Industrialization of Digital Operations

This combination of a global delivery factory that offers strong people and process, a powerful platform, and decoupling plus specialization allows creative agencies to do what they do best, in concert with brand teams, and design great campaigns that are then funneled through a single hub to be rapidly built, regionalized/customized, and delivered on a global scale at enormous production savings, typically up to 40%. Speed to market increases at three to four times what companies not leveraging this model can achieve (see Figure 4.20).

As a best practice, people and processes are put in place to ensure compliance with brand standards as well as digital and technical and quality standards. This is critical when companies are working, as many large pharmaceutical companies do, with many different agencies

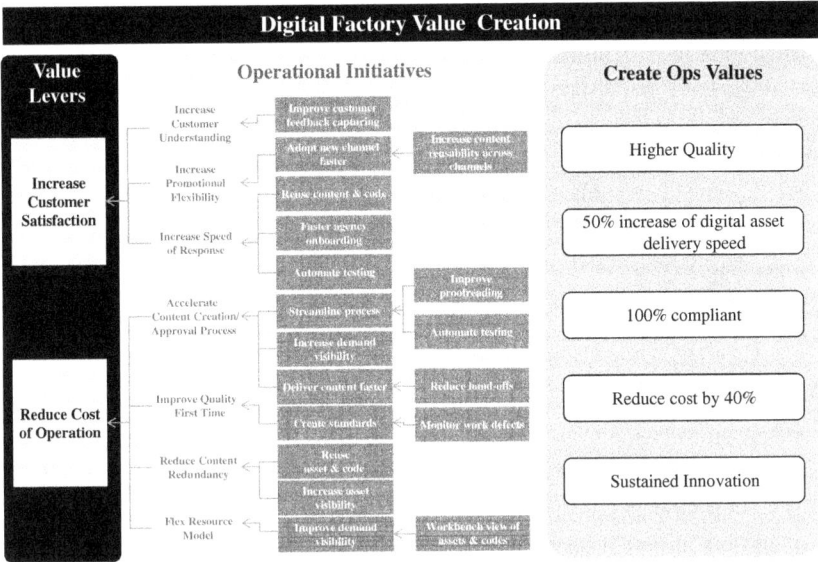

FIGURE 4.20   Digital Factory value map.

around the world. Well-structured digital factories enforce brand and style guidelines, development and architecture standards, management of metadata and taxonomies to ensure data and assets are well organized, and have rigorous compliance and quality assurance processes. One of the significant efficiencies that we see coming from this rigor is large cost savings coming from the reuse of digital assets. Often, when a company employs many agencies, creative teams are unaware of exactly what digital assets a company already owns. These can include photography, video, graphics and audio files that can be very expensive to create or buy a license to use. This becomes even more complex when global marketing mixes with local marketing. There was one case where a business had been consistently spending over USD 1 million per year on photo shoots, all of which were essentially of the same thing, just being done by many, many agencies around the world for various local campaigns. The factory model, and its digital platform, leverage Digital Asset Management systems and the processes necessary to ensure a company's digital assets are organized in a way that makes locating them and reusing them simple. It also enforces the policy of potential asset reuse as a first option, rather than always opting for creating brand new assets unnecessarily. The amount of reuse that is germane for each company varies; but, in the pharmaceutical sector digital asset reuse typically accounts for an annual 25% reduction in the cost of production.

The fully formed digital factory and platform that is rapidly gaining prevalence in the pharmaceutical industry is at last bringing the benefits we marketers had hoped for years ago to light. Their design is indeed complex and not to be taken lightly, but as is almost always the case, it is very difficult to design something that, on the surface, appears incredibly simple. These models require companies to be "all in" to gain the full benefits, in the sense that they are ready to build robust digital platforms, build strong collaborative partnerships with all their digital marketing vendors, and create global processes that continuously drive forward effectiveness, efficiency, and value. This requires not only commitment, but flexibility on the part of all involved to look at performance across the entire digital ecosystem, inside and out, and be ready to adapt to forever changing technology, market shifts, demand and strategies.

The final output of a fully operational global digital marketing operation such as this is powerful, but has plenty of room to grow. As smart organizations adopt and refine this model, the immediate gains in speed and cost reduction will be equaled by further gains in revenue and margin maximization. All the pieces of the digital puzzle are in place to allow marketers to interact with each customer on more of a one-to-one basis than ever before on a global scale. The companies that can pull all this together will be at the forefront of digital marketing and put significant distance between themselves and any lagging competitors.

This part of the chapter was co-authored with Jeremy Pincus and Kevin Nicholas. Jeremy is a digital strategist and an evangelist of digital industrialization and is currently with GlaxoSmithKline. Kevin is a digital and mobile guru with many years of digital marketing and mobile solutions strategy and execution experience across various industries. He currently works with Infosys.

SCREAM WITH MOUTH SHUT: GLOBAL COMPLIANCE STRATEGY

The first half of 2012 had record-breaking regulatory fines, USD 6.6 billion in total. The year ended with the highest fine given in a single year—USD 9.8 billion. In July 2012, the US Department of Justice announced that GlaxoSmithKline (GSK) had agreed to pay USD 3 billion in criminal and civil fines for its misdeeds in inappropriately marketing Paxil and another antidepressant, Wellbutrin; The fine was the largest ever healthcare fraud settlement imposed by the US on a pharmaceutical company and settled both civil and criminal charges. The company had downplayed safety risks and promoted products for "off label" uses that were not medically accepted indications covered by federal healthcare programs. GSK conducted several double-blind, placebo-controlled clinical trials that ran between 1994 and 2001 to establish Paxil efficacy in adolescent depression [35] but it never established the endpoint. There are several other large fines, including Pfizer (a USD 2.3 billion settlement in 2009), Abbott (a USD 2.3 billion settlement in 2012), Lilly (a USD 1.4 billion settlement in 2009), Johnson and Johnson (a USD 1.1 billion settlement in 2012) and many more [36]. These fines are for off-label selling, wrong claims, and non-compliant marketing and sales practices.

The pressure on pharmaceutical quality and compliance functions is increasing significantly with regulators taking a more aggressive approach to inspection, establishing bigger budgets and becoming very keen on enforcement. The regulators' shift is influenced by the dissatisfaction of patients with product safety and constant underperformance of products as opposed to their claimed benefits. Health authorities across the globe are becoming more vigilant and are increasingly listening to the patient.

With the huge responsibility of healthcare carried by a pharmaceutical company, it absolutely needs to behave like an important stakeholder—it can't just look at the company's profitability but must take responsibility for improving society's well-being. The pharmaceutical industry has done so much for humankind but is constantly attracting media attention for the wrong reasons. The most prominent discussions are about drug safety issues, lack of fair pricing, data disclosure issues, marketing problems, DTC advertising spend, ethical issues around animal and human testing, illegal promotion and detailing of drugs, and lately, pharmaceutical fraud. The list is already long and is getting longer. Pharmaceutical companies are under enormous pressure to tackle these issues.

The pharmaceutical industry is being pressurised to go for smaller clinical trial-based product approval to bring in products faster and cheaper to satisfy a demand that is not being met. There is a great opportunity for pharmaceutical companies to help patients in long-term care, but this can only happen if the industry behaves in a mature fashion and does not influence product upsell. And there are many more similar opportunities. Is the industry ready to take more responsibility? May be not.

In early 2012, Novartis suspended production at a plant in Lincoln, Nebraska, where various over the counter and animal health medications are made. There were several consumer complaints of foreign products found in its solid-dosage form of medicines. This has not only hurt Novartis's reputation but also created a shortage of the supply of other products to the consumers. The direct financial impact of similar quality issues can be substantial. Though Novartis's plant closure cost is not disclosed, closing a plant to fix a quality problem can cost over USD 100 million and recalling a batch of product can cost USD 10 million or more. This spend includes consulting costs, facility improvement, costs for keeping the facility idle and penalties for failing to supply product to customers.

The non-compliance has severe indirect effects too—high-profile product failures and recalls, fines, plant shutdowns and audits make investors, healthcare professionals and consumers nervous; it drives doctors and patients away; and it cuts sales and tarnishes the company's image.

While the industry is aware of these consequences and how serious they are, it faces several challenges. One challenge is the individual quality process which is relatively simple, but the overall effectiveness of a quality and compliance system relies on complex interactions between hundreds of separate activities, and a considerable amount of human judgment, often made by various internal and external company partners, making the decision-making even more complex. The failure of a single process or of a single interface between processes can have profound consequences on both the quality of product and/or compliance. Pharmaceutical business is changing fast and the regulatory requirements are as well. The business epicenter is shifting to that of the emerging markets to change the regulatory complexities. Patients have become more informed through the use of the internet and are more concerned about their treatment options. There has been an increase in outsourcing, and vendors and partners are playing a bigger role in end to end drug development and the launch process. Patients are increasingly concerned about product safety and benefits—they have become more demanding. Thus the regulators have become much better at cracking down on non-compliant operations.

So how should the pharmaceutical industry respond? In this new era of compliance, the industry is asking the health authorities several questions in order to improve compliance:

- Who should handle compliance? Will individual business units handle it or would it be under centralized regulatory governance? As governance has always been a major non-compliance point, will regulators provide better guidance on this issue?
- My customers are well educated and well connected through social media. How can I take part in this without violating complex regulatory needs?

- How do we handle a fast moving pharmaceutical business model—brand focus changes, organization structure changes and business shifts in newer geographies? More powerful global health authorities have several new regulations. Decades ago it was a US dominated compliance process. Europe, Japan and Australia then joined the decision-making process in the second wave. Today, the pharmaceutical industry needs to work with over 60 different authorities to manage a successful global brand.
- Some compliance guidelines are hard to follow in today's world. They are also time-consuming and expensive, for instance the FDA wanting live monitoring of speaker programs in order to ensure compliance. Will the FDA allow video- or tele-monitoring instead?
- Regulations are increasing every day, whether it is EVMPD or IDMP or Product Track & Trace. Will more regulations reduce the problem of non-compliance?
- What is the trade-off between regulatory mandates and operating freedom to the pharmaceutical industry? While advising a top global pharmaceutical company on their patient compliance strategy, I found several conflicting issues between the pharmaceutical manufacturer, patient and regulators. The manufacturer wants to go beyond selling the pills; they want to provide additional support to keep the long-term care patient motivated to take medication regularly. This needs constant communication with the patients through various means—phone, SMS, website, etc. But regulators don't allow free communication between the manufacturer and the patient as this could influence the patient's product choice; they also want the manufacturer to report any adverse events that may come out during this communication. Although pharmaceutical manufacturers want to help patients, their hands are tied and they need to be careful with every communication. To avoid too many adverse events, the manufacturers restrict their communication and don't provide the option of free text patient feedback. Instead, they give them the drop-down—a fixed menu option to provide feedback. This definitely restricts the freedom a patient may want to have while communicating with a product manufacturer. This is a unique situation where all three parties want to help each other but can't do much within the regulatory restrictions. To provide better support to the patient, manufacturers should be restricted less in their communication with patients and healthcare professionals. Health authorities should rely on the manufacturer's corporate ethics and can monitor their behavior through inspections and reports.

There are many more questions that need to be answered to create the right global compliance and quality structure. While the industry may have several questions, they still need to have a strategy in place to operate in full compliance with a global strategy and country level implementations to comply with local health authorities.

Pharmaceutical compliance is far-reaching and complex but there's a common trend. The top spots in the Food & Drug Administration (FDA) observations (FDA 483) list has almost permanently been taken by Corrective and Preventive Action (CAPA), Document and Records Management, and Management Controls. This reiterates the fact that the industry needs to focus increasingly on content (document, art, video, etc.) management and establish the governance model to ensure compliant operation.

There are a number of documents that are created for internal operations and some are created to submit to the health authorities. The external submissions include IND (Investigational New Drug), NDA (New Drug Application), BLA, etc. that are focused on R&D function; manufacturing and manufacturing R&D creates ANDA (Abbreviated New Drug Application), OSHA (Occupational Health & Safety), W&M (Weights & Measures), CAPA (Corrective And Preventive Action), SPL (Serialized Product Labeling), etc.; Sales and Marketing creates promotional content and aggregate state reports and many more.

There are various other functions, e.g. Outcomes Research, Medical, Legal and Finance, that are responsible for benefit comparison, product safety reporting, pricing-benefit strategy and health outcomes reports. This is a representative set and not complete; some functions also vary from one organization to another and from one location to another. But my target is to discuss a solution which can easily be modified to suit specific needs of a company and address most of the issues around content management. The content of each of these submissions follows a specific protocol. They all follow the basic activity blocks of "create-review-approve", "publish and submit", "track" and "strategize and plan" (see Figure 4.21). This is the basic cycle of content management that can potentially come under regulatory audits. Let me take an example the DMF (drug master file) which gets submitted to regulatory authority in connection with an application, e.g. NDA or ANDA. This document has its own life cycle—it gets created during the application and needs annual report submission to keep it active. Pages in the document cannot be dropped once submitted and all modifications to the original should be separately produced. The life cycle involves several stakeholders across various functional areas within the company and their external partners, e.g. the contract research organization (CRO) or contract manufacturing organization (CMO).

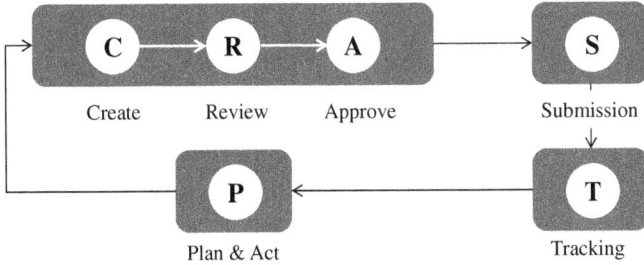

FIGURE 4.21 Regulatory submission creation.

If we do a persona-based analysis of stakeholders involved in the DMF life cycle using a model, GRIP, the following model can emerge: GRIP = goal, responsibilities, input needed and pain points.

The chart in Figure 4.22 shows the involvement of Regulatory Affairs, R&D, Manufacturing, QC and other stakeholders to accomplish the goal of error-free DMF submission. While this goal has been chosen by one stakeholder, Regulatory Affairs in this example, other stakeholders may have their own goals that in combination will help to achieve the final goal. It's important to separate these goals that are specific to a stakeholder to create more focus. This focus will help to establish responsibilities specific to their own goals, which will then ask for the right input from other teams, creating a collaborative work environment. The work may come with pain points that need to be addressed for improved output and better compliance. I have used the GRIP framework to analyze specific functional areas to create a persona-based working model. This

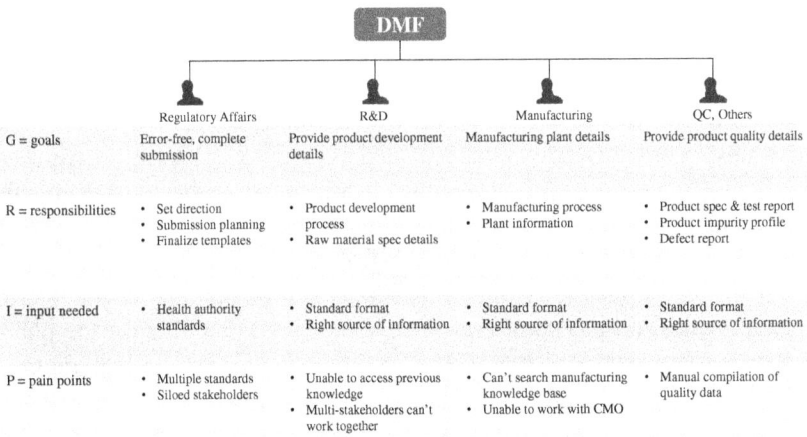

FIGURE 4.22 Stakeholders in DMF creation.

helps in the right segregation of duties and to create a collaborative work environment to accomplish overall business goals.

Now, if we do a GRIP analysis for another submission document, say for the NDA, you will find many similarities. The process, the player, the input, the output and also technology needs are similar. There are common pain points as well. This creates an enormous opportunity to streamline the regulatory content management function. The operations can be shared and a shared services operating model can bring in several benefits to an organization.

> *Standardize.* Process, stakeholder and technology system standardization can eliminate re-work up to 50%. This also makes the solution future-proof with potential organization changes, M&A and brand acquisition from other organizations.
>
> *Collaborate.* With the partners and vendors playing a bigger role, a technology solution to bring all the teams, including internal and external stakeholders, onto a single platform will greatly increase the efficiency of the submission process. The challenge remains in bringing these stakeholders together, navigating through the security issues and bringing in significant cultural changes.
>
> *Reuse.* Effective reuse of content from earlier submissions, using part of the existing content instead of rewriting it entirely can speed up the submission process significantly. This aspect has always been downplayed by the pharmaceutical industry whereas other industries did this many years ago. This is a wake-up call for Pharma. Technology solutions on auto-population of metadata and content, and auto-correction of errors based on past submissions can definitely help.
>
> *Comply.* Surprisingly, regulatory submissions are not error-free. Over 60% of submissions to the health authorities are erroneous or submitted with insufficient information and are put on legal hold. I have heard frustrated business leaders lament: "Why can't we submit information of our own innovations the way the FDA wants us to?" It significantly adds to the time it all takes to get it to the market if the submission is not right the first time. Tracking submissions, end to end traceability, re-submissions, and responding to the health authorities, on time and error-free every time, can all save the pharmaceutical companies millions of dollars and cut several months from the approval time.
>
> *Analyze and improve.* Regulations across the globe are evolving too fast. Compliance operations, e.g. submissions, need to be constantly updated with these changes, especially at country level, to refine

operations. Health authorities do welcome feedback for improvement at their end, which is generally overlooked by the pharmaceutical industry but can be achieved through a well-organized shared services model as it helps keep track of everything, analyzing it and measuring improvements.

If we setup a single metric to measure regulatory compliance success, it would be 'high level of transparency'. Health authorities all over the world will look for traceability of events—from submission documents to individual reports to analytical data and analytical methods, etc. A company with the highest level of transparency will gain customers' trust. This level of transparency not only responds to a request from the health authorities but also proactively shares reports and events with all stakeholders. It can be achieved by using smart technologies in a regulatory content-shared service operating model. However, there are far too many technologies on the market and they need to be handpicked carefully. Most solutions do not provide end to end capabilities that manage regulatory submissions for the various functions in a company and can be scaled to suit global needs. The regulatory compliance solution may consist of a process framework, people strengths, governance model, health authority change monitors and a robust technology platform to back it up to support easier execution of regulatory submissions globally.

The solution given in Figure 4.23 consists of vertical and horizontal services. The vertical elements are Strategy and Plan, Create, Review, Approve, Submission and Track. These vertical business functions are

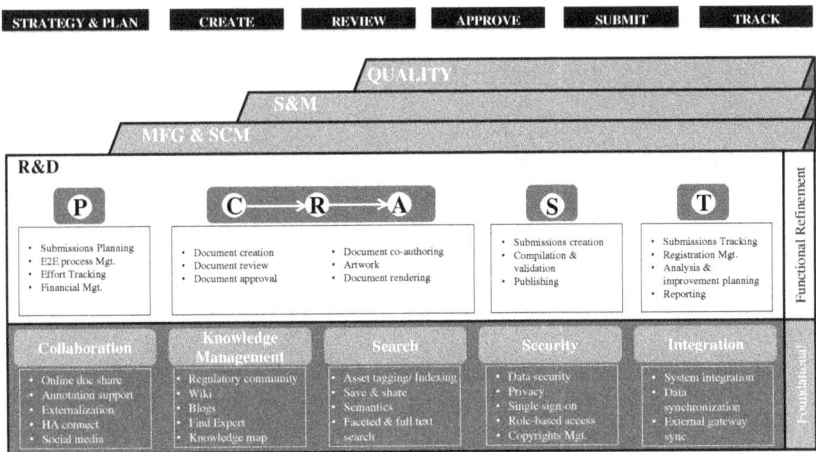

FIGURE 4.23   Compliance submission platform architecture.

delivered with horizontal functions such as Collaboration, Knowledge Management, Search, Security and Integration forming the foundation.

Strategy and Plan. What, why, who and how are the critical questions that need to be answered at the beginning of a submission project. A team of experts and analysts works together to create a strong planning foundation for submission of a product in a market. I recommend that we look at the historical data, including similar products in a different market, different products in a market, earlier submission of the same product in the same market, and submissions with the same external stakeholder, to make the submission strategy more successful. I strongly suggest that we revisit the strategy frequently during the entire submission life cycle for better outcomes.

Plan. The planning helps steer a project and helps us to reach the final goal. We need to build in auto-planning of tasks, notification of movement between tasks or on slippage, and impact assessment in case of regulatory change, which will all enable the business team to get a clear view on the impact it will have on the timeline and help them meet the plan.

Create. Template management, metadata management, virtual document management, linking documents, document translation, working on different file formats—though the list of operations under creation is long, this is the function where multiple stakeholders work on collecting and putting the content generated from different teams into the required format and build the base for a submission.

Review. The content authoring process is so complex and runs through so many different hands that review of the content becomes highly critical. Some of the features, e.g. ability to capture the comments, consolidate, interactively allow the author to respond, track changes, offline review, and ability to comment on other reviewers' comments, will be crucial.

Approve. As discussed above, any unresolved issues in the submission documents will put the overall submission on hold. It is therefore critical that the submission goes through a review and a stringent approval process. The approver should be able to approve the documents at different stages and levels and finally eSign it. The create, review and approval process is cyclical and continues till the reviewers and approvers are finally satisfied that the submission is complete and ready.

Submission. Once the submission is approved it needs to go through a submission validation and publishing process. As part of the validation, a system check is done to ensure that submission complies with the health authority requirement, that a compliance report is generated, and that errors are identified and auto-corrected wherever possible. This can also be done for interim versions to speed up the process. For the second part of the publishing system, submission-ready composite documents are created. This will create links and convert the documents to the required formats. After this, submissions are stored in the appropriate file share from where they get submitted, either manually or electronically, to the health authorities.

Tracking. Tracking is all about managing the product information during the product development life cycle process. The various submissions for each product are tracked at many health authorities. It maintains the end to end traceability of each submission. I always propose that the interactions and queries received from health authorities are interactively managed. An excellent alert and notification mechanism, and complete traceability of records at every level will not only allow the industry to respond to queries quickly but accurately as well.

Collaboration. Increasing the footprint and the role the external stakeholders play is becoming highly critical for pharmaceutical companies to get them to play a bigger role in regulatory submission as well. This solution will enable externalization of the regulatory submission platform, online co-authoring and review. Topping it off with strong social media features like blogging, sharing, chat, etc. will create just the right recipe for an efficient submission process.

Knowledge Management. Each organization and all its business functions generate a huge volume of data. This data contains a wealth of information and should be used effectively. Through knowledge management we want to introduce reuse functionality (auto-population of metadata and content), guided authoring, auto-correction or suggestion of errors (based on past data or queries received from health authorities), etc. This functionality would not only reduce the number of queries from health authorities but also reduce the overall time taken for submission.

Search. This function is getting redefined across the board. It is about getting the right information at the right time in the minimum amount of time. The technology solution to make this effective by leveraging semantics and ontology will make the regulatory affairs users effective and powerful.

Security. With externalization, security will become a highly critical function. Through this component, appropriate controls will need to be established to ensure data privacy, security, unauthorized access control, copyright management, IP management, etc. Hosting the solution on a Cloud needs further extensive secured controls. Pharmaceutical industry is moving towards it and I myself know a lot of nonprofit organizations are investing in it while working on new technology solutions. I have personally experienced setting up a secure control environment to host R&D applications on a Cloud.

Integration. I was astonished when I saw the number of applications used by a leading pharmaceutical company to support the regulatory affairs operations. It is high time we look at consolidating and integrating all these applications. In these complex operating environments it is critical that all the business functions are aware of the status, issues and challenges. Integrating all the critical applications and delivering them completely as a single solution will provide a strong foundation for the next generation solution.

The most important aspect of bringing in a new solution successfully is not just changing the process or changing technology. It is all about new ways of working. The people aspect supercedes all other strategies and this needs to happen at multiple levels—Compliance team (Regulatory Affairs), Information management team, external partners and all internal functional areas. Some of the people strategies worked well:

- Early adopter—find an early adopter who becomes the champion of change
- Build relationships—compliance is seen as policing and better impact can be achieved only through tighter relationships between compliance and other functional areas—R&D, Manufacturing, Field Sales, Marketing, etc. Other functions should view this as a supporting business unit and not a policing unit trying to find faults.
- Senior leader certification—senior leader support is eminent but I propose senior leader training and certification on compliance needs. This makes them accountable for compliance acts and their support comes more naturally
- Compliance everywhere—compliance personnel should have "a seat at the table" in other business meetings, such as sales leadership convention, manufacturing planning, R&D pipeline reviews, etc. This helps embed compliance needs early in the functional plans
- Compliance anytime—constant communication and messaging to other business units to update them on policies and to inform them about new or upcoming policies. This helps to predict future challenges and proactive action

- Information accessibility and conduct—easy access to employees through web-based systems
- Controlled strategy—with faster and easier access to information, messages can be spread across controlled boundaries if the proper measure is established. Social media has created lots of opportunities but poses several compliance challenges as well. Compliance strategy needs to establish boundaries.

In the new era of pay for performance, the submission documents need to be written even more carefully and should most likely be re-written several times. The regulators will be far more watchful and pharmaceutical companies will go through a lot more scrutiny, not only during the approval process but constantly as they compare their brand performance with the claims they have made. A robust submission solution with the right technology as its foundation is the only way forward.

Pharmaceutical compliance plays a much bigger role than simply keeping the company compliant by ensuring the right submission—it helps improve a company's image to the external world. This helps shape the company's mindset towards improving healthcare and giving back more to the society. Some of the best practices of compliance are:

- Make the right claims based on clinical data analysis: do not exaggerate product benefits and safety profiles. Make a business plan as per the product claims and not based on the off-label sales
- Set the right price—don't ask for a higher price just because you don't have much competition and you have spent a good amount of money on R&D and continue to have a large spend on marketing. The public thinks the industry wastes money on advertising—think about the patient's well-being and how many people can't afford the medicines you produce just because they are priced at a level beyond their reach. Assess the cost–benefit ratio of treatments and decide whether a drug should really be priced that high
- Think of the patient—don't do anything that will eliminate the possibility of better or cheaper alternatives. The product exclusivity extension is one such example where the inventor tries to extend their exclusivity for as long as possible. This is counter-intuitive for better healthcare
- Sales and marketing practices are areas of potential misdemeanor in several areas including providing gifts to HCPs, any incentives to physicians and off-label drug promotion. As the primary interface between the manufacturing companies and patients, physicians and other healthcare providers, the sales and marketing teams need to take more social responsibility about meeting sales targets.

Create more awareness about the compliance needs, training and re-training of all the stakeholders in the entire product ecosystem to have a much more positive impact on society as a whole.

WHY PATIENTS CONTINUE WITH MEDICINE: PATIENT ADHERENCE

It's springtime and Michele is driving through the countryside on the US east coast. Trees in bud and beautiful flowers in bloom make her roll down her windows to enjoy the weather. Little does she realize just how much pollen is prevalent at the moment and, soon enough, she starts sneezing, gets a runny nose and even has difficulty swallowing her coffee when she stops for a break. She starts having difficulty in breathing and her overall body stress has aggravated her blood pressure. But she still has to drive 150 miles before she reaches home to get help.

The situation will change tomorrow though when pharmaceutical companies, medical devices companies, healthcare providers, caregivers and technology companies all come together to improve overall healthcare beyond just selling their products. They will have joined hands to provide innovative healthcare which will take care of patient needs end to end, or prevent the patient from falling ill in the first place.

If I hypothetically connect the few innovations already available today, Michele won't have to go through the suffering while enjoying her beautiful drive through nature.

With the advancement of mobile technologies, Michele's allergic condition can very well be taken care of without much suffering. This is an integrated care model—all the stakeholders in the caregiver ecosystem quickly come together to help the patient (see Figure 4.24). Early in

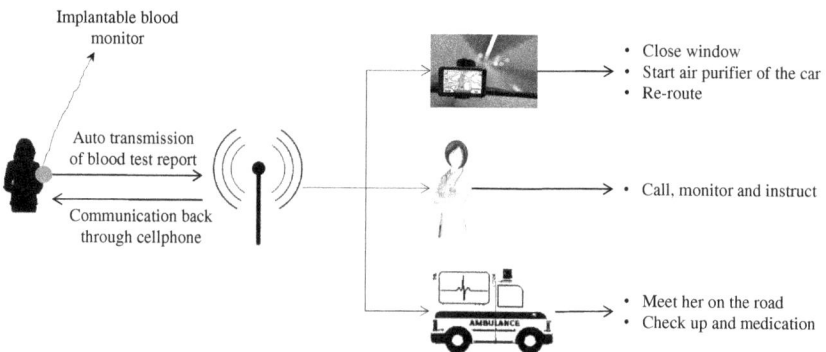

FIGURE 4.24   Patient treatment on the go.

2013 researchers at Ecole Polytechnique Federale de Lausanne (EPFL) in Switzerland developed an implantable blood monitor [37]. A smart blood monitor can measure the allergen-specific antibodies and send the signal through Michele's smartphone to her GPS system in the car she is driving, her physician, and to a local healthcare provider. The GPS system immediately rolls all the windows up, starts the car air purification system and recalculates her route with lesser pollen counts. The physician's office makes a call to Michele, checks her condition and provides instructions. The local healthcare provider comes in on the same call and with specific instructions from Michele's physician, plans an immediate check-up en-route. Michele's condition is taken care of within 10 minutes.

This may sound futuristic but I strongly believe it's closer than we think. All the components either already exist or are in the development cycle which will be available within the next couple of years. This solution needs both the pharmaceutical manufacturer and the payers to make it complete. But every stakeholder in this chain is working with others to make this possible. This is what I describe as an end to end health solution beyond just the selling of products. If Michele is taken care of in this way, I can confidently say she won't leave this health network and will continue with the medication as needed. She will comply on her own and won't need to be pressurized to continue with the medication regime. The combination of stakeholder willingness to improve the patient experience and technology progress will help patients to adhere to medication.

Poor adherence to prescription medications and treatments has been labeled a "worldwide problem of striking magnitude" (World Health Organization, 2003) [38]. Compliance to medication falls below 50% after the first six months of long-term care, oncology and lifestyle drugs; over 30% fail to refill prescriptions as they feel better after the initial start of their medication. And this is not about financial hardship alone—financial incentives have been proven to have only limited effect in changing patient behavior.

Research suggests that a high-touch approach is required in modifying patient behavior to comply with the medication. Today, highly educated patients who research disease conditions and are well aware of treatment options can't just be motivated by product safety and benefit stories. Thus, adherence interventions require a very good understanding of patient behavior, health beliefs, and a sound technological approach to adjust the solution to the patient's day to day regime. It should be easy to use and much more beneficial to the patients.

When we worked with a top pharmaceutical company to create a compliance program for one of their brands which needed a continuous medication routine of four months, the greatest success came with introducing a smartphone-based registration process. The entire process consisted of four major steps—buying the medicine, registration to the program, following the program mandate and analyzing progress. All registered patients got personalized care on disease education, instructions, reminders and monitoring of their improvement through an online portal. The pharmaceutical manufacturer also set up a call center for those patients who didn't want to use the web portal; some patients also used SMS technology to connect with the company for any support they wanted. The web portal had the capability to build a "patient diary" for the entire duration of the medication which included information about the patient, motivational stories, improvements made and projecting their benefits against the benchmark of other patients. There were options for personal interventions with the pharmaceutical company if the patient wanted to make it more personalized.

Our analysis showed the program was highly effective and it increased the patient cure ratio by 20%. The patient cure was only about 27% for the patients who didn't enroll in the program; it went up to 47% for the people who enrolled in the adherence program. So, the program was hugely successful. But a bigger problem was to attract patients to the program. We introduced a mobile device-based registration process to eliminate some of the registration barriers which we discovered during interviewing patients, including [lack of] internet connectivity at home, keeping the receipt till registration is done, etc. We introduced a smartphone application to scan the product receipt bar code to enter into the web portal. Patients had to agree to the terms and conditions to register. They could return in their own time to modify their profile if needed. This increased patient registration by 87% and proved the point again that if the adherence program is very easy to use and the patient's everyday routine stays the same, the program might become very successful.

Patient compliance can be improved significantly through increased personal and non-personal interventions. Hence, there is a need for a platform that can bring patients, physicians, payers and the pharmaceutical manufacturer together to create a better healthcare environment (see Figure 4.25). Patients need the education, motivation and personal touch, physicians want to cure and pharmaceutical companies want to be directly associated with a larger healthcare community which can provide easy access to the information that can help patients and physicians.

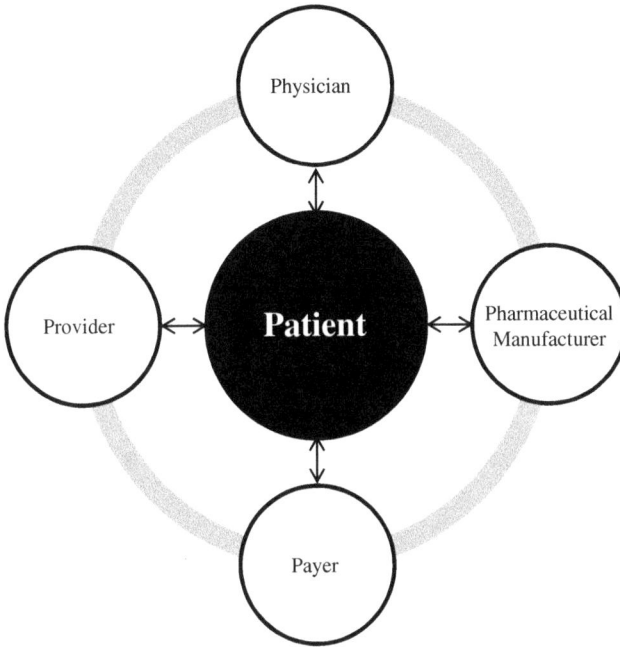

FIGURE 4.25   Health & wellness ecosystem.

The ubiquity of technology and the openness in sharing and gathering knowledge has brought in a drastic change in the way patients view disease management. Patients are becoming more proactive in managing their health and are making use of technology to find out more about their disease, diagnostic and therapy options. Today, over 80% of patients take some action based on online information on therapy, products and physician selection. The binary communications between physician and patients or physician and pharmaceutical manufacturers need a common ground to share, care, educate, monitor and cure for better healthcare. A technology-driven solution can create significant value for all the stakeholders. It can also influence the pay for performance process and can ensure pharmaceutical manufacturers receive payment for their product.

An adherence solution can benefit pharmaceutical companies significantly. Patient non-compliance to prescription contributes to about 15% revenue loss for the pharmaceutical industry. A revenue uplift can be achieved by providing extra support to the patients and physicians through the adherence programs (see Figure 4.26). The model I have recommended to several companies is called EIRMA—Educate, Instruct, Remind, Monitor and Alert (see Figure 4.27). The adherence

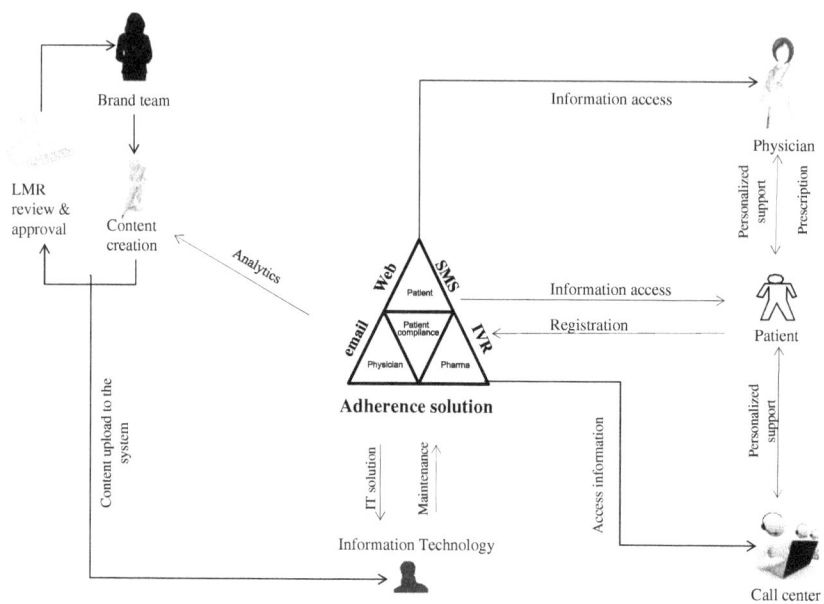

FIGURE 4.26 Patient adherence solution.

solution can support patients with all these services to improve medication compliance.

Educate. Increases product knowledge, safety, benefit and risks. This helps increase knowledge of the disease, symptoms, causes and medication options.

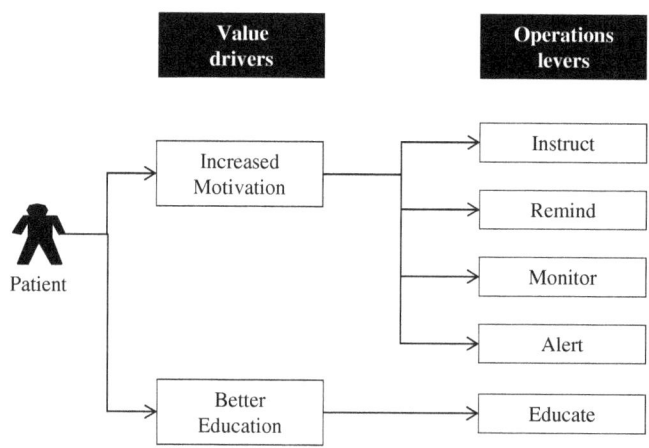

FIGURE 4.27 Patient adherence solution.

Instruct. Medication process details, events-based action as per the patient preferences in the profile, and inform about next steps as per the medication courses.

Remind. This initiates a reminder for medicine intake, physician visits, supplementary care activities, and task completion status.

Monitor. This can collect patient data, check patients' progress against benchmarks and track behavioral changes.

Alert. Notifies specific people as per the patient preferences in case of special events, alerts stakeholders at the end of milestones, send alerts for any side effects.

I had recommended building a standard infrastructure, also known as a platform, to create this solution which can be reused across various different programs. The biggest challenge for a brand team is to fit the adherence program development timeline within their campaign plan. A traditional technology project takes a long time if it is built from the ground up. Hence, a platform-based approach will help by reusing approximately 60% of the marketing and technology assets and using the remaining 40% effort to customize it and make it brand-specific. This shorter timeline will fit well within the brand's campaign time frame. There are several components that can be reused:

- Method to analyze product pipeline to find the patient compliance program fitment
- Mini business case including ROI analysis
- Compliance assessment framework
- End to end, multi-party program management method
- Success criteria—pre-built KPI and reports.

Table 4.1 gives more detail on other reusable technology component details.

Offering an adherence solution along with the medicine will not only help improve the overall health of the patient, it also helps differentiate the product in the market. A specialty pharmaceutical product with a caregiver service attracts a much better price than a product without, and can eliminate competition. The healthcare reform will push the product price downward and payers will always look for better justification of the medicine price. I'm very certain that the product benefits on their own will never be enough to attract the price a pharmaceutical company would look for. Interestingly, while the US market is yet to establish the pay for performance model, there are several European countries already following the practice. One such example is the reference pricing model

TABLE 4.1

Standard Components	Standard Templates
Registration Bar code validation Segmentation Profiling Channel Integration (SMS, IVR, email, etc.) Fulfillment Company style guide, logo External partner interfaces: call center, agency, content developer Analytics packages Secure HCP registration Emails: username confirmation, forgot password, opt-out, auto-reply and standard day or profile-based emails Calendar, diary Search	Content display based on program day Content display based on user input Reminder rules Alert rules Profile-based display—user experience Reports—program uptake, usage, profile, success Compliance input and tracker Communication preferences

Basic Data Structure	
• Patient profile • Program type • User inputs	• Survey response • Aggregate calculations • Call center activity

in Germany. Germany requires pharmaceutical companies to demonstrate the added therapeutic benefit of a new drug in comparison with the available treatment alternatives. The manufacturer has the potential to negotiate a better price with the health insurers after one year of market access if they can prove the additional benefits. Belgium and France are two other countries following a similar model and many other countries are in the process of following suit, including the UK. The patient adherence programs could prove the additional benefits.

Providing room for customization depending on the target audience, cost benefits and geographic requirements has always been appreciated by the brand teams, as the ROI is often not easy to articulate. A platform-based solution with well-defined values including a standardized process and systems, faster time to market and low cost implementation can make it real. The industry needs this solution for the benefit of patients, physicians, providers and the manufacturing companies and it should be an essential component in any brand campaign.

THE PERKS IN EMERGING MARKETS: GO GLOBAL

The quality of treatments and medicines will determine the choice, the country where it came from will not. The global economy will normalize the healthcare options and pharmaceutical market very soon. The highly educated patient community today cannot be misled by the manufacturing locations' driven premium prices. We, the patients, cannot afford the inflated cost of healthcare and the significant prescription drug cost component any more. What patients want will make emerging markets more attractive to a pharmaceutical manufacturer.

Patients have already chosen to use generics more, which has resulted in a greater increase in product manufacturing in the emerging markets than in the developed markets. The healthcare situation in emerging markets makes this market even more attractive. The middle classes who have jobs and access to healthcare in the emerging markets will nearly double to approximately 3.2 billion in the next five years. This will increase the medicine consumption in the emerging markets to 30% of the world pharmaceutical market demand.

The use of generics in the developed market is increasing every year. The current prescription pattern in the US shows an 84% use of generics and it is predicted to grow significantly in the next couple of years. The constant price pressure in the developed countries will make the generics even more attractive.

The evolving health insurance market in the emerging economy will open the doors for branded products as well. Patients and caregivers will be more open to even higher priced product options if insurance companies support them. However, the branded drug market will undoubtedly create a significantly lower impact in comparison to generics. Branded products need to be localized with a lower price tag to remain competitive in this market.

All these drivers, along with more favorable government policies and the increased growth in per capita healthcare cost have made the growth in emerging markets far greater than in developed markets. The growth in emerging markets is projected to be 12–15%, whereas developed markets are projected at 0–4% in the near future.

The term "emerging market" is used to describe developing nations such as India, Brazil and China, which are in the process of rapidly growing or becoming industrialized. In many ways, it is a misleading term that fails to represent the importance and influence that many of these countries already hold in the global economy. In reality, emerging markets have already emerged and pharmaceutical companies in particular

	TODAY	2017
Market size	20%	30%
Target population	1.8 Billion	3.2 Billion
Per capita spend on healthcare	+	+++
Government policies	Protective	Favorable
CAGR	14%	12-15%

FIGURE 4.28   Emerging market growth.

have already taken confident steps towards establishing themselves in the region; for example, pharmaceutical brands in established countries, such as Novartis and Pfizer, have already invested in R&D facilities, sales forces and administrative operations to India and China. Pharmaceutical companies spent over USD 20 billion in the emerging markets in 2012, up by 75% from 2011. Most pharmaceutical companies in the matured markets are establishing themselves solidly in the emerging markets.

The chart in Figure 4.28 describes the value drivers for the pharmaceutical manufacturers to move into emerging markets. The average growth projections for all large pharmaceutical companies are as high as 25% in 2015. While this is a very ambitious growth target, they are yet to have all the pieces of the puzzle together. To me, there are five themes that can help pharmaceutical companies reach their targets.

Create a Personalized Market

Two factors will drive the pharmaceutical market in the emerging economy over the next five years. The first is more access to healthcare for a larger part of the population; the second is that the disease profile will tend to match that of the developed countries. Taking India as an example, about 780 million people in India today do not have proper access to healthcare. The situation is changing rapidly and this number is expected to drop to 20% by 2020. This shift will increase the population who can afford healthcare to 540 million and the population increase will add another 75 million who can afford healthcare to take the overall target population over a billion. Other emerging markets have a similar situation. In Brazil, for example, 32 million people have moved into the "middle" and "high" income brackets during the last five years, and that figure is expected to double in the next five [39]. This rapid growth in the target population for the pharmaceutical companies will increase the growth of the market significantly.

The disease profile in the emerging markets is being leveled with the developed countries. Cardiovascular disease, diabetes and cancer are the most prevalent disease conditions causing death, even in these emerging markets. This creates an opportunity for the large pharmaceutical companies to bring in their specialized products for these areas as they are available in the matured markets. These products may need country specific innovations before marketing. One such example is to innovate heat resistant packaging material for a sensitive product, as India lacks the cold chain distribution availability. The combination of bringing in innovative products and making them available within the infrastructure boundaries and the price limits can help create a personalized market for a company. Roche's decision to bring in a "local version" of a cancer drug at a significantly lower price than that was available on the market is the best example of creating a personalized market for long-term value creation.

Knowing a country's market can also happen through acquisition and partnerships. Abbott Pharma's acquisition of Piramal's generics business in India, and the Roche partnership with Emcure are two strategic examples.

Demystify the Local Supply Chain

The biggest challenge for a big pharmaceutical company in the emerging markets is to understand the local supply chain and make it useful. The supply chain system in emerging markets is very different from one country to another. Some countries are far too fragmented and have complex drug supply networks. India has about a million stakeholders in the pharmaceutical product supply chain including distributors, stockists, sub-stockists and small shops that can sell medical products (see Figure 4.29). The complex network completely shields a manufacturer from what is really happening in the market. The manufacturer doesn't get product visibility through this multi-layered, manually managed network with its non-standard processes and near-zero data integration. This makes the distribution system ineffective and very long. No visibility causes disproportionate product stocks in the market and impacts the order processes. A manufacturer in the matured markets is used to working with a much simplified supply chain with very low numbers of distributors and will need to go through a significant learning curve when setting up in a country in the emerging markets.

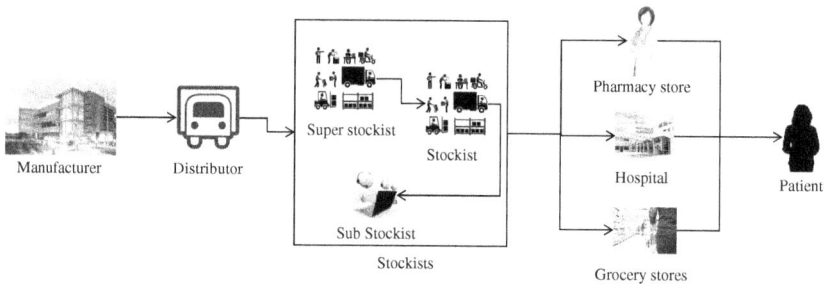

FIGURE 4.29 Emerging market supply chain.

Trade-Off Volume and Price

In early 2013, Roche decided to reduce their cancer drug price in India by 30%. The company decided to drop the price of Trastuzumab by 31% and the price of Rituximab by 53%. These are reductions on the existing drug prices in the country. If compared with the US market, these prices are about 10% of the drug prices in the US. How will Roche be able to meet these prices and still make a profit? The answer lies with local manufacturing. Roche has an agreement with Emcure Pharmaceutical to manufacture these Roche products for the emerging markets. They defined this as being the localized version of the same products.

Reducing the price of the drugs in the emerging markets will still make sense in the long run. Drug consumption per capita in the emerging markets is 10–20 times lower than the US or other matured markets. Cardiovascular drug per capita consumption in the US is 193, whereas it is only 15 in the emerging markets. Drug consumption can therefore go up by 10 times within the existing target population, as improvement in the economy in many countries means they can afford more medicine. The new target population will be doubled by 2020. This means Roche can potentially increase the drug sell by 40 times within the next few years. The trade-off between price and volume is worth the risk. The local manufacturer produces the product at a lower cost, which makes the business still profitable.

There are several other companies including Pfizer, Novartis, GSK and BMS who are looking at moving into emerging markets with their branded drugs.

Value-Added Services to Patients

The disease profile in the emerging markets indicates the rising occurrence of chronic disease. Patient adherence programs benefit patients with chronic diseases significantly. As described in `Why patients continue with medicine: Patient Adherence' section, a product with the adherence program attached can differentiate it in the market.

Adopt a Friendship Model

The majority of western pharmaceutical companies would struggle to compete with local businesses as they lack the "home advantage" of understanding the intricacies of the market. That aside, they do have the strength of being able to provide financial investment and global expertise that can't be rivaled by the smaller competitors. Rather than competing for the same patch, large pharmaceutical companies should build local business relationships and make themselves part of a country's core healthcare ecosystem. A well-defined, local, empowered and integrated key account management structure can help streamline this ecosystem and be more effective. This needs a strong focus in building the right local team with a long-term focus [40]. The GlaxoSmithKline (GSK) operating model in India is a good example of how long-term planning can create significant value for the company. GSK never changed their local presence even after the policy in the country changed to make the market less compelling. However, they continued their business with a focus on vaccines, in-licensing and partnerships to make them one of the largest western companies in India.

Several significant challenges such as the patent law, drug licensing and data exclusivity issues have crippled the emerging market for several years making it unattractive for the large branded drug manufacturers. Gaining approval for new products in countries in the emerging markets compared with those in developed markets takes much longer. The approval time in Russia takes up to 18 months longer than the US and three years longer in China. Large pharmaceutical companies also prefer not to perform Phase 1 clinical trials in India or China because their data exclusivity is not stringent enough. Brazil does not have any explicit data exclusivity regulations as of now.

In India, the patent office ruled against the intellectual property rights for several prominent drugs including Pfizer's Sutent, Bayer's Nexavar, Novartis's Glivec, and Roche's Tarceva. There are several situations for large pharmaceutical companies to introduce a branded drug in India including the enforcement of compulsory licensing.

Emerging markets are risky across the board with respect to legal and regulatory issues, the labor market, tax policy, security, political stability and infrastructure. However, many countries in the emerging markets use technology very effectively to minimize certain risks. One such example is to adopt a connected supply chain model through a single technology platform which can connect distributors, integrate the sales force, connect stores for order capture and analyze all data to improve visibility across the chain for the manufacturer to plan the production and supply efficiently. This platform uses various channels to connect with the stakeholders—web portal, SMS and call centers.

A well-conceived orientation to the latest market trends combined with localization strategy will help large pharmaceutical companies success in the emerging markets. All big pharmaceutical companies need to be part of the emerging markets' growth today or tomorrow—so an early start will create a stronger foundation. The new product strategy, partnerships and local acquisitions help to establish a newcomer, but a long-term strategy with serious commitment to the growth of the country can make the difference.

Chapter 5

Measuring Business Values and Success

THE PHARMA VALUE CYCLE: HOW TO REDEFINE STAKEHOLDER VALUES

The pharmaceutical industry needs multiple shots in the arm to treat its "anemia". Its anemic growth, margin, and its inability to take care of its stakeholders need treatment. The current state of affairs is very grim. The industry isn't growing as much in the matured market, the debt to equity ratio has doubled in recent years, and over 40% of pharmaceutical employees are very confused. How can the healthcare industry improve without treating these issues first? The prognosis is that the industry is not creating enough value for its stakeholders—customers, employees and shareholders.

I see diminishing stakeholder values in financial, relational and social aspects. Many companies have been successful in creating value for their customers but they haven't had a mechanism to protect it long-term. The initial value creation is easy as it's a new beginning with a superior financial status; however, diminishing value needs to be avoided through long-term value focus which needs better stakeholder relationships and the promise of greater social value.

The 3-3-3 model of Value Cycle in Figure 5.1 identifies three core stakeholder groups at a pharmaceutical company. They are the customers, employees and shareholders. If we assign a value expectation to each of them, we get a total of three value expectations by the core stakeholder group. Employees want rewards on commitments they make towards their company, customers want better value for their money, and shareholders want the best return on their investment. Each of these values consists of three value dimensions—financial, relational and social. A long-term bond between a company and its stakeholders needs all these dimensions—a missing component weakens the bonding. This is the

Pharma's Prescription. http://dx.doi.org/10.1016/B978-0-12-407662-4.00005-2

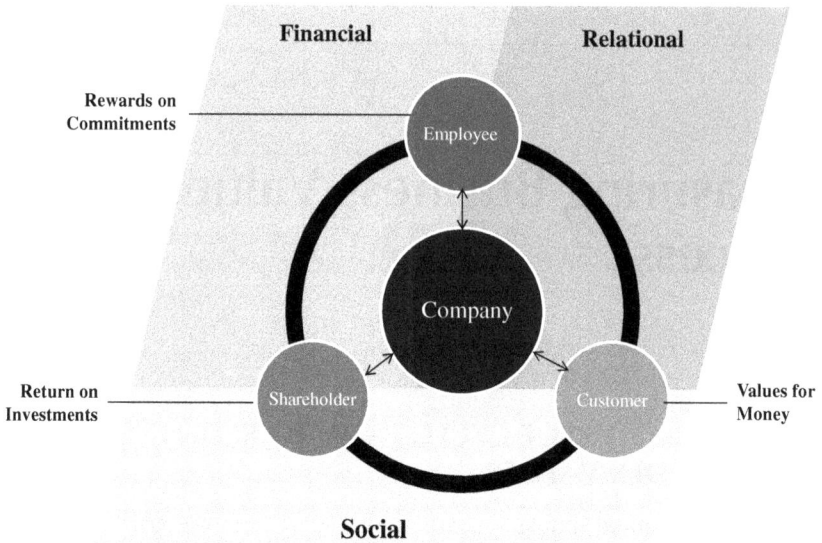

FIGURE 5.1 Core stakeholder groups and values.

"value design" of an organization in the 3-3-3 model. As its name tells us, this model describes three stakeholders, three core values and three value elements in the corporate value cycle.

The "value design" phase is followed by the "value creation" phase which looks for answers to the following questions:

• What three changes will you implement to make the plan work?
• What three milestones will you establish to monitor and track progress?
• What three investments will you make to make this happen?

Pharmaco Inc. (not its real name) is a global company with operations in 22 countries and over 20,000 employees. As a start-up company, it delivered more than the market expectations and has set very high stakeholder expectations. After a period of time the company is still doing well but is unable to constantly deliver the stakeholder values at the same level it did at the beginning. There's nothing really wrong with the company except that it's unable to grow as fast as it did before when it was small. The market, however, wants the same level of return it produced in the beginning and reacts badly every time the company announces its results. In one such year when the company showed no growth and failed to meet the market expectation, it lost significant market capitalization. While the company leadership was undecided on its course correction, they needed to make a quick decision—what value would it create for their employees?

The company executives had to increase their focus on the customers. They tried to find a differentiated product and decided to make some financial trade-offs between the product price and profit margin expectations as a short-term measure. Their decision was based on increasing the cash flow and providing much better value to customers. They feared losing customers fast if they failed to create differentiated values within a short time. So, the company's top priority was to take care of its customers.

The shareholders were nervous as the market had reacted negatively. Company executives know well that shareholders never wait for more than a year or so if the return on investment does not meet their expectations. So, the company leaders had an easy decision to make—their shareholders needed better care.

The compromise therefore had to be with the employees. A recent survey by an external consulting company showed that over 40% of their employees were confused with their work, career direction, values they create for the company and the rewards they receive from the company. An even scarier finding was that most of this group of employees had spent over five years with the company. Five years is a landmark number for the employee stickiness quotient. It shows that most employees in this group have done well for several years and are a real asset for the organization. They have got to know the values of the organization well, know what the company offers, have been the brand ambassador of the company and have created value for the customers over several years. However, they haven't received the right value from the company. The stickiness quotient (over five years of employment) indicates they have established a good relationship with the employers. Have they received good financial benefits? Have they got the right social value? Probably not. This is evident from the "worry factor" assessment in the pharmaceutical industry. Over 60% of employees felt worried about their job— they fear losing their job even though they have performed well. They were even more worried about the unfair performance evaluation and unsatisfactory relationship with their managers. So, the combination of lower market excitement, unclear financial decisions and negative social and relational factors has left a large number of employees confused.

The management had the same pie to distribute into three parts. Customers and shareholders have got the bigger pieces—employees came in last. I think this shows very traditional decision-making and no boldness in leadership decisions. They go even further down the traditional route when the employee pie gets distributed disproportionately amongst various employee seniority levels. To understand the employee situation better, let's divide the employee groups into various levels—junior with less than five years' tenure with the company, middle with less than five years with the company, middle with over five years with the company, senior executives and very senior executives. In difficult times, many of the senior groups come together to take the company out of danger—that's true leadership. The very senior group expects the seniors to take this responsibility without expecting much benefits (mainly financial) in return for the promise that they will be taken care of in better times. The junior groups need to be benefited in real-time or else they will move on for better opportunities outside the company. The very senior group also makes decisions favoring their well-being, unless they are under a great deal of external pressure. So the most affected groups are the middle and senior level employees. These two groups have spent enough years with the company, have made up their mind on skill areas, are looking towards building their specific business acumen and are very less likely to make any drastic moves. This is again traditional middle to senior management career decision-making, i.e. looking for stability over anything else. A lot of the time, this behavior is exploited by the company leadership to give the middle to senior management the smallest share of the pie.

A great company should differentiate by taking a different approach in sharing the benefits across various employee groups. The 3-3-3 × 3-3-3 model of "design values" and "create values" for the stakeholders is described in Figure 5.2. Values for the company are devised by the "design values" module–customer, value is defined as "values for money", employee value is defined as "rewards on commitment" and shareholder values are defined as "return on investment".

Once values are defined, each stakeholder group will have three value elements that will help deliver overall values for the group. The "values for money" segment in the customer group has three value levers—better therapy, continuous support and better price. Pharmaceutical company customers, for instance patients, would rate a company highly if it manufactures and delivers a better quality product which cures patients. They also want constant support from the company to help by educating patients on their disease condition, or a complex support to monitor a chronic patient condition. Obviously no one wants to pay more for the improved benefits and they expect an enhanced quality product as well

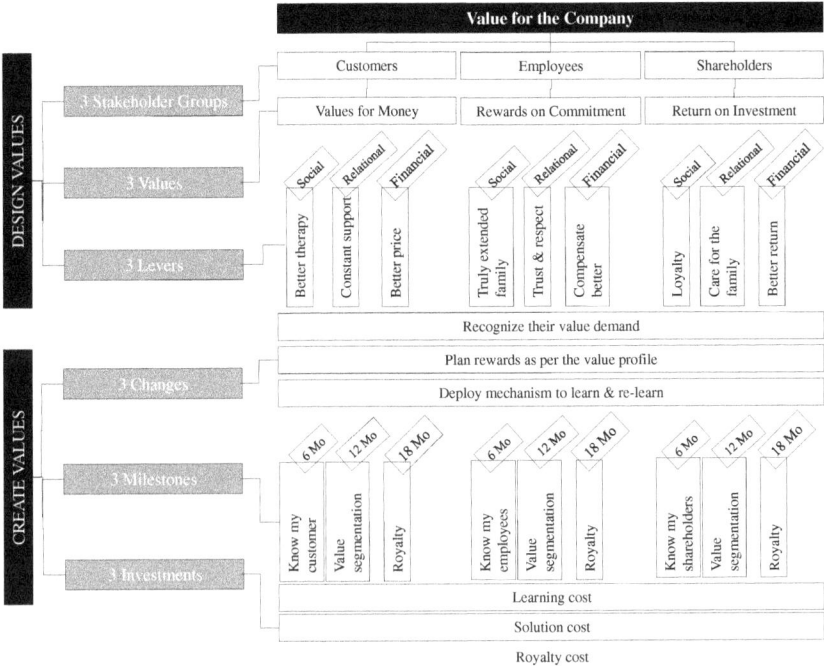

FIGURE 5.2   Value design model.

as support at the same price if not lower, to increase patient satisfaction with the pharmaceutical company. These value levers need to be customized for a specific stakeholder group, and may be aimed at a specific stakeholder within a group—for example, the value levers for patients may be different from that for physicians, although they belong to the same customer group.

Once values are designed, the next step is to give exact details on how to create values by making operational changes. The "create values" segment starts with deciding on making three changes across stakeholder groups or for a specific stakeholder. The examples of changes I have listed in the model are "recognize their value demand", "plan rewards as per the value profile" and "deploy mechanism to learn & re-learn stakeholders better". The value demand can be recognized during the learning process and a specific plan can be created to reward as per the demand. It's very important to learn about the stakeholder value demand again and again as it changes from time to time. The next step is to create three milestones to monitor and track the progress of the value creation. The milestones can be tracked in two different ways of which one could be timeline-based—for example 6 months, 12 months and 18 months. The progress can be tracked as "how well you know your stakeholder needs", "can you create values based on the stakeholder segmentation", or "can you share loyalties as per stakeholder contribution". These are just examples of various milestones and you need to create your own based on company preferences and measurement culture.

No strategy can work without making an implementation plan. No plan works without making an investment. The investment doesn't necessarily need to be monetary investment but it can be investment of time, investment in monitoring and tracking, providing infrastructure, investment in change management, etc. The investment plan needs to cover the process, people mindset, and technology. Knowing your stakeholders comes with a price—implementation of the model costs money and a solution to create value costs money. Finally, a loyal stakeholder needs to be rewarded with royalties, which costs money as well. But this can't be seen just from the cost side alone. If implemented, this model can create significant value to the company, including revenue growth, margin improvement, brand value enhancement, and marketing and sales costs reduction as loyal customers spread the good news through social networking, etc. I have personally experienced several value design and implementation opportunities, where pharmaceutical companies could increase customer retention significantly through implementing focused value creation initiatives.

Financial strength has huge power in keeping the core stakeholders together. Increased cash flow, higher revenue and better margins create much more flexibility for the company's management team to keep everyone happy. It is important to understand the financial value in everything we do in a business set-up. The next section shows one such example in a shared services organization.

THE UNBEARABLE FINANCIALS: MODELS TO REALIZE FINANCIAL VALUE

As the pharmaceutical industry redefines its core operations, a large set of business functions are being executed through external partnerships. This helps pharmaceutical organizations to leverage a greater skills base without having to invest in building those capabilities in-house. It also creates the flexibility of refining the operations faster. However, this operating model comes with a big question mark—where do I get the fund to change the operating model and how do I ensure the model will pay back quickly?

A large number of organizations have embarked on initiatives to move their entire business or a part of their business to operate in a shared services model. While many have enjoyed great success by creating significant financial values, several have struggled to design and manage such a transformation. One of the key reasons for failure is the lack of an appropriate and transparent financial model to design, implement, monitor and report the shared services financials.

This chapter will focus on creating the right financial model, starting with an executable business case and a constant focus to realize the benefits in the operations. However, it's important to understand some of the basic pillars of a shared services operation in which the financial model can be executed.

If implemented correctly, an IT shared services model can create significant values for a pharmaceutical company, not only reducing cost, but creating a self-funded innovation model. Some pharmaceutical companies that have embarked on shared services in the last few years have achieved the desired operational maturity, and a saving of up to 60% depending on their level of maturity [41]. How did they do it?

The first step is to determine the changes to bring in through the shared services by understanding the existing services available to the users. While working with several large pharmaceutical companies I have realized that most business operations work with a diverse set of service providers with no clear definition of services, processes and financial transparency. This creates lack of standardization, unclear accountability, almost zero measurement of success or failure and lack of cost-visibility. If this is the situation you are working in, you have an excellent opportunity to improve operations and reduce cost through a centralized delivery model. This model ensures end to end service delivery as per predefined service level agreement and cost structure by services used.

As the new service model enhances value to the organization and its customers it's important to establish a value model which consists of designing value metrics during the design phase, monitoring them during operations and reporting the realized values to all the shared services stakeholders. A shared services operation can produce savings by eliminating redundancy in operations, staff, and process steps and by delivering services from low cost locations. So you need to build a financial model which captures all these elements. This chapter will help build the model in a step by step process.

Firstly, let's define a few personas (actors) in a business situation (see Figure 5.3) where the shared services will be established.

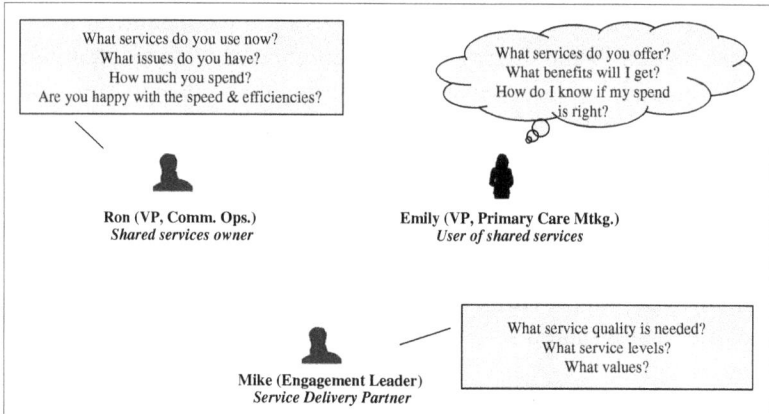

FIGURE 5.3   Shares services personas.

Ron, the VP of commercial operations, wants to consolidate marketing operations across various brands globally. He also wants global partners to deliver services locally. Let's call him the owner of the shared services.

Emily, the VP of primary care marketing, supports Ron's marketing operation centralization initiative as it would improve marketing operations' productivity and reduce her operating costs. She is the user of Ron's shared services.

Mike, the service delivery executive, works with Ron and Emily to define the shared services and financial models. He is the delivery partner.

While Ron builds this end to end shared services (let's call it Global Services Operation) it will be used by Emily. As the service user, Emily wants all services to be delivered consistently with the right quality, on time, on value and at a lower cost. Ron needs to design the shared services keeping Emily's expectations in mind and Mike needs to ensure meeting those delivery expectations.

A good service model always puts the user perspectives at the center—in this case, let's see the model through Emily's eyes. In the pre-shared services model Emily has been using a discrete, project by project delivery model with a price tag attached to each project. She will now evaluate the following aspects before adopting the new delivery model:

• What services will you deliver? Will you deliver a part of my business function, for example a campaign management service, or just a task within the campaign management, for example, testing the content before its delivery to the end users?

- How do I know your price is reasonable and justified?
- How would you distribute the shared services cost across various brands if I manage budgets by brand?
- How will you align your price with my budget? It's financially easier to compare spend if you deliver the entire business function, but how will I reconcile it if you deliver only a part?
- How will you ensure continuous improvement and bring in new ideas into the service delivery to avoid business and technology obsolescence?
- I don't have very clear visibility of the number of campaigns we will run for the year. I may not run any campaign for some months but several campaigns may run simultaneously in another month. How will you handle the fluctuating demands?
- I don't want to box myself into a permanent cost structure without knowing much about your pricing model. What flexibility will you provide to fine-tune the financial model based on historical data?
- My marketing content production price varies by region and by country. As shared services is a global function how will you meet my price expectations locally at each market?

A customer-centric global shared services organization needs to address all of these questions raised in Emily's mind. Knowing user needs and understanding their current financial management structure is the first step to building the new model.

Financial modeling in a shared services organization involves foundational levers such as demand visibility, demand seasonality, budget structures, invoice management, centralized funds, chargebacks to brands and adequate reporting. These levers may need tweaks to be unique to an organization but the major construct doesn't change. This model works on four basic principles—Simple, Reasonable, Predictable and Beneficial (SRPB).

Simple: Ron and Mike discussed and agreed that anything that is difficult to understand is not worth implementing as a process. The goal is to present the cost of the service to the service users in a simple form—it should be similar to a utility bill which shows the services used, the unit price and the total cost for the service. This should also provide the usage trends over a time period to alert the users on their spending pattern. This can be achieved if services are defined at a much more granular level and each component is priced independently to proportionate cost as per the usage. In Emily's case, Ron and Mike have itemized the digital content price of the lower units including creative, production, test, release, metadata, library management, localization and regulatory packages. Each of these service units is then further classified based on their complexities. A price tag needs to be created at the smaller unit level so that Emily can choose her service and calculate the total price for herself as she uses various services. This is a pay as you go model.

Reasonable: A shared services model reduces the operation cost significantly and users expect a lower price tag. Mike works closely with Ron and Emily on the following aspects to create a reasonable price tag for the services:

1. Sharing a skill between projects can reduce the cost per project significantly. This can be done through proper planning and working on demand and predict work volume. Using skills across various projects with over 80% utilization brings down the project cost by up to 25%, in comparison to execution of a stand-alone project.
2. Location plays a big role. If a task can be done from outside your company, it can be done from anywhere. Choose low cost delivery locations.
3. Stringent service levels and a compressed delivery timeline can cause havoc with the overall price. My advice is to not create stringent service levels for non-critical services. Plan early to avoid a last minute rush and pay more to deliver within the timeline.
4. Users no longer pay more for higher quality. Quality is a basic expectation today and should be factored into the base price.
5. Regulations, security, data privacy and business continuity should be taken very seriously but local level controls need to be established. Local implementation will help to localize the price instead of applying a compliance price tag across all projects globally. These are highly debated points and create significant barriers in global shared services operations and very often significantly increase the price. Address them upfront and communicate with the stakeholders for better acceptance of the controls needed.

Predictable: Predictability of quality service delivery, delivery speed, price and compliance should be assured through the service design. Service user satisfaction is directly proportional to the predictability of the service. User confidence in the delivery service will come with time as the shared services adjust to the variability of business demands. If we look at the example of the campaign management again we see that this is dependent on competitive market situations, brand performance, regulatory needs and also the local market situation. Campaigns are designed, based on these variables and the same service price per campaign is harder to commit to. But the shared services should be able to build on a knowledge base over a period of time to fine-tune pricing models by predicting various campaign situations and pricing them appropriately upfront. Brand teams love this price predictability as it takes a major task out of their to-do list.

The cost of not being able to predict prices reasonably well in advance is so high that most organizations today penalize their executives for budget inaccuracy. So the financial model should have the ability to estimate the price at a higher level of accuracy and, most importantly, should be able to adjust to the demand uncertainty. The financial model should have clearly defined boundaries for changes in volume, service levels, stakeholder mix, locations and more.

Beneficial: This is by far the most ignored aspect of the financial model. The purpose of creating the shared services is to provide business benefits—cost savings, increased speed to market, higher consumer satisfaction, better innovation and more. Most importantly this model should be able to produce actual dollar savings that can be returned to the corporation or used as an innovation fund to improve operations. This is the basis for building a self-funded shared services innovation model. But over 80% of the shared services do not have any mechanism to constantly measure business value and show the savings realization. They may define it in the beginning but it never measures up to or compares with the planned numbers. A shared services organization cannot constantly improve without value realization. Financial data needs to be collected, analyzed and refined to constantly optimize service delivery prices.

Now that Mike has established the basic design principles, he will work on the process to design and implement the financial model. He follows a very simple process (see Figure 5.4) to create, test on a pilot scale, implement and optimize the model.

This is a simple process used in most service roll-outs. However, this process needs to be customized for a specific shared services model for a better result. Here are those specifics that worked in Mike's situation.

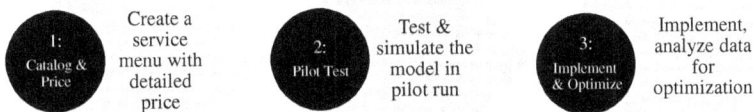

FIGURE 5.4   Shares services personas.

STEP 1: Create a Detailed Service Catalog and Price Point

The key is to define a service catalog that works for all the stakeholders in every situation. Emily's needs may change for various business situations—she may need end to end support for some projects but may need to use shared services only for one or two tasks of the entire project. Mike's service menu should be flexible enough to meet Emily's varied needs. However, Mike needs to make sure his services are well defined with the right scope boundary, dependencies on the other teams, expected inputs and outputs. As the shared service may not responsible for the entire project delivery, Mike needs to ensure his part of the service is protected from any project issues outside his delivery scope and control.

A skill-based breakdown of various services makes shared services a flexible enough operation for Emily to work with multiple partners if needed. This flexibility in working together with multiple partners with specialized skills helps mitigate any business risks during start-up of a shared service. So the financial model should be able to adjust costs based on services split between partners.

A web channel-based campaign will have campaign planning, customer segmentation, marketing storyboarding, layout design, content development, testing, metadata tagging for analytics, production release and the FDA (for the US market) submission (see Figure 5.5). Ron and Mike need to price these services independently to increase financial transparency and create flexibility to use multiple partners who are specialized in each service line.

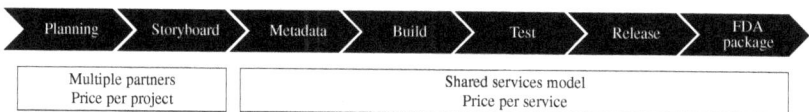

FIGURE 5.5   Shares services personas.

The component-based pricing is important as the pharmaceutical IT project delivery has not been impressive. Data shows that only a little over 50% functionality gets delivered to the end users through a turnkey project, over 80% of projects go through a time extension, and the same percentage that goes through projects overrun. The key reason for this failure is not having confidence in estimating the timeline and the cost. My experience shows that breaking a project into multiple parts with input and output clearly defined in each part creates much more clarity for confident estimation. I have validated and used this model at various pharmaceutical companies—it worked everywhere and has become very popular.

The pricing model can be more accurate if some fundamentals are kept in mind—(a) to have good knowledge about the service, (b) to know the parameters that would influence time and cost of delivery, (c) to understand price variance based on service levels, if any and (d) the benefit of delivering all services together.

The diagram in Figure 5.6 is representative of pricing parameters in an eDetail presentation development.

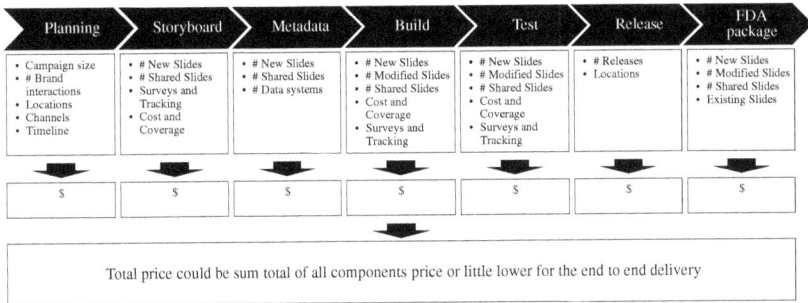

Planning	Storyboard	Metadata	Build	Test	Release	FDA package
• Campaign size • # Brand interactions • Locations • Channels • Timeline	• # New Slides • # Shared Slides • Surveys and Tracking • Cost and Coverage	• # New Slides • # Shared Slides • # Data systems	• # New Slides • # Modified Slides • # Shared Slides • Cost and Coverage • Surveys and Tracking	• # New Slides • # Modified Slides • # Shared Slides • Cost and Coverage • Surveys and Tracking	• # Releases • Locations	• # New Slides • # Modified Slides • # Shared Slides • Existing Slides
$	$	$	$	$	$	$

Total price could be sum total of all components price or little lower for the end to end delivery

FIGURE 5.6 Pricing elements for eDetail content development.

Service levels can have a great impact on the delivery price for some services, for instance web development and brand site maintenance. The pricing model for a website in Figure 5.7 has components that are time dependent. If delivery needs to be rushed for business reasons the operation may ask for a premium service price. Creating multiple options and clearly communicating pros and cons with the end users keeps them happy and ensures everything stays financially beneficial.

A content build can be expedited by adding additional bandwidth to the project team and by enabling multiple parallel work streams, but it may increase the build cost. It's important to identify the common services that can be shared across various projects. The cost of these services needs to be attributed to individual services based on the complexity,

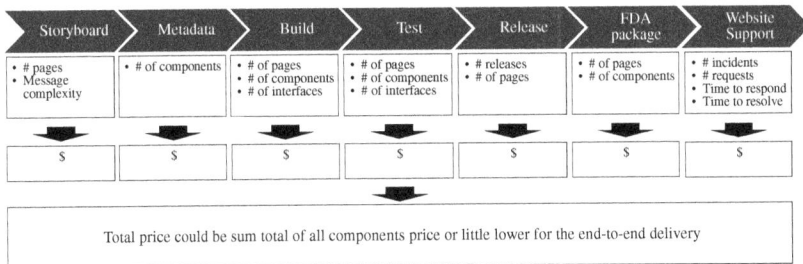

Storyboard	Metadata	Build	Test	Release	FDA package	Website Support
• # pages • Message complexity	• # of components	• # of pages • # of components • # of interfaces	• # of pages • # of components • # of interfaces	• # releases • # of pages	• # of pages • # of components	• # incidents • # requests • Time to respond • Time to resolve
$	$	$	$	$	$	$

Total price could be sum total of all components price or little lower for the end-to-end delivery

FIGURE 5.7 Pricing elements for Web content development.

skills required and effort spent. For example, an efficient execution will need effective stakeholder management, demand management, planning discussions with business, project management, compliance management and governance that need to be distributed across various services. My experience tells me that some over-investment in this user interaction area can only be beneficial. Service users want to understand how their work is being done—they want to remain connected and well-informed via this front-ending service team. The initial estimation of this team can be done based on the number of business stakeholder interactions, the number of brands to be supported, the number of locations and their geography, the number of time zones to be supported and the number of creative agencies with whom to interact. This team, together with service users, can optimize delivery and cost as service delivery matures. I recommend not shying away from investing in this area even if the overall price looks higher in the beginning. There could be requirements for using systems and tools that need to be allocated proportionately. Create a simple algorithm to attribute these costs to the individual services—the commonly used techniques are to create a shared fund for this or to distribute it in proportion to the effort spent in performing in each project.

It's very common in the industry to execute an end to end project through multiple partners based on their expertise. Create a delivery model where multiple partners can deliver parts of services. Emily won't have to deal with too much change management if she doesn't need to replace too many existing delivery partners. Campaign planning and storyboarding at times are very specialized and Emily may need external companies to help. If Mike's team can work with these external companies and receive inputs for his web development or eDetail work it's a win-win situation for all. Mike will then provide build, test and release services. It may happen that the company's regulatory team wants to manage the FDA package creation and submission and they won't want Mike to provide this service. Mike's output becomes the input for the regulatory team. So, in this situation there are three parties involved to execute the campaign design and development. This is only to plan and create a campaign and excludes campaign analytics and monitoring services where other partners may be involved.

The most critical aspect in working with multiple stakeholders is to define standards that are useful to all partners. While everyone does their bit they need to ensure the output is usable by the next partner without any challenges and this is possible only when all stakeholders use predefined standards. As the owner of the shared services, Ron has to

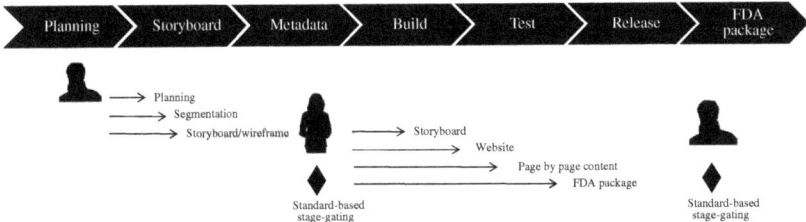

FIGURE 5.8   Pricing elements for Web content development.

ensure end to end processes are defined with working standards and hand-off protocols.

A standard-based gating process at each handover makes the delivery seamless (see Figure 5.8). This also ensures excellent traceability for any errors. The best model is to define the standard, using checklists to receive the input from another team and rejecting it at the point of entry if not delivered as per quality.

STEP 2: Pricing Model Simulation Through a Pilot

Mike's pricing model is based on various attributes that can change based on task complexities or changes over a period of time as delivery matures. So, the pricing model needs to be simulated through constant monitoring of data. This can be done by creating a longer list of levers that control the pricing attributes. For example, the primary attribute of "a number of pages" for a website has simple, medium and complex levers. These levers can assign weightage to a primary attribute. A complex page will require more effort than a simple page hence more weightage will be given to the complexity over "a number of pages". So, Mike needs to monitor these attributes and levers and adjust them as his service delivery matures. My experience always tells me to start with the simplest model and go more complex, only to fine-tune the price over time—no model is perfect on day one.

Mike's pricing model is now ready to use in projects. He can select how many projects he wants to use to gather data for model refinement. It's important to allow several months for the monitoring of certain attributes before making any changes.

Refine boundary conditions: a shared service becomes most efficient through sharing skills across various projects and functions. This needs a steady flow of work in the system. Boundary conditions need to be set for minimum work volume, maximum work volume, service level changes across brands, a service demand profile—a combination of only one service versus all services versus a few services, and more. All will have an impact on price optimization.

Process conditions: check for process overloads or no process chaos. Both can jeopardize efficiency and, if rectified, can add much to the pricing optimization. Right balance is needed to excel the service delivery and user satisfaction.

Time adjustments: this can add significantly to the overall time line and cost in a multi-partner situation. Each team can add their own timeline with certain buffers factored into it. All of them combined increases the overall time. Some extra bandwidth to monitor all partner activities and timelines can help optimize the price further—the extra bandwidth will be time well spent.

STEP 3: Implement and Optimize

As the model is piloted successfully, Mike can now roll this out to all the projects in the shared services model. He now has experience of using a simple pricing tool with service needs, skills, effort and boundary conditions adjusted to the price more efficiently. This tool can generate cost details for the brand managers based on the services they have consumed and tells them what's going to be on their invoice. Mike can produce a trend report with services used, service type, cost, etc., very similar to the utility-based pricing we discussed at the beginning.

Mike now needs to focus on creating a benchmark, either by analyzing prior data points, most of which are not available in the exact form he would need, or by keeping track of the projects he executed. The data-driven approach helps keep the end user community much more convinced.

Constant connection with the end users is imperative. Monthly governance reports and invoice trend reports do help. It is also necessary to become sensitive to the evolving needs of the brands—additional channels, geographies, languages—and to adjust services periodically to meet these needs. Over a period of time, once all the stakeholders are satisfied with their data, Mike can focus more on reviewing opportunities for continuous improvement. The opportunities for improvement go beyond the shared services operation, and involve notifying Emily's team on potential improvement including brand communication, messaging, channel decisions, and content improvement.

Value Realization

If designed correctly, I have never seen a shared services operating model failed. I have designed and implemented several of them with big global pharmaceutical companies, and have witnessed huge benefits. These benefits go beyond the initial cost saving. The money saved can contribute significantly to boost the innovation engine of an organization, which at times runs slowly because of the lack of dedicated fund availability. The savings in operation is exponentially proportional to increase in innovation power. If you can save 30% in operations and return 50% of the savings to the corporation, the remaining amount can increase the innovation capacity by over 100%. This is a very powerful benefit that can be obtained by using a shared services operating model.

References

[1a] Making Counterfeiting Unprofitable. http://www.sproxil.com/blog/; Accessed 7/4/2013.

[1b] Organovo creates living, three-dimensional human tissue models. http://www.organovo.com/3d-human-tissues; Accessed 6/20/2013.

[2] The Use of Medicines in the United States. Review of 2011 IMS Health. April 2012.

[3] Key Facts About Prescription Drug Costs. http://pharma.org/sites/default/files/pdf/KeyFactsAboutPrescriptionDrugCostsMay2013.pdf; Accessed 5/24/2013.

[4] Open innovation. http://www.15inno.com/2012/08/09/oicrowdexamples/; Accessed 7/8/2013.

[5] www.FDA.gov.

[6a]–[6b] www.news.bbc.co.uk.

[7] Use of big data in research. http://www.microsoft.com/casestudies/Windows-Azure/Molplex/Aiming-to-Deliver-New-Drugs-Faster-at-Less-Cost-in-the-Cloud/710000001667; Accessed 7/6/2013.

[8] www.clinicaltrials.gov.

[9] www.uic.edu.

[10] en.wikipedia.org.

[11] Bosch ME. Recent advances in analytical determination of thalidomide and its metabolites. Journal of Pharmaceutical and Biomedical Analysis 2008; 0107.

[12] www.cdisc.org.

[13] http://www.lifescienceleader.com/magazine/past-issues3/item/4363-pfizer-perseveres-in-pioneering-virtual-clinical-trials?list=n.

[14] Lab integrations. http://apps.thermoscientific.com/media/CORP2/CONNECTS_Irish_DA_REVISED.pdf; Accessed 5/31/2013.

[15] Paperless lab. http://www.lifescienceleader.com/magazine/past-issues3/item/3767-two-companies-two-new-paperless-labs; Accessed 3/31/2013.

[16] www.supplychainmanagement.in.

[17] www.En.wikipedia.org.

[18] Pollen monitoring. http://www.claritin.ca/en/claritin-mobile; Accessed on 3/31/2013.

[19] Human Error Reduction. http://www.fdanews.com/store/product/detail?productId=30732; Accessed on 3/31/2013.

[20] CAPA monitoring. http://www.pharmamanufacturing.com/articles/2004/233.html; Accessed 2/21/2013.

[21] http://www.tugportal.com/Portals/_default/UC11NA/9A%20-%20Achieving%20ROI%20and%20Realizing%20Benefits%20with%20TW.pdf; Accessed 3/31/2013.

[22] www.accountingtools.com.

[23] www.infosys.com.

[24] http://www.mckinsey.com/insights/business_technology/delivering_large-scale_it_projects_on_time_on_budget_and_on_value.

[25] http://www.fda.gov/iceci/inspections/inspectionguides/ucm074875.htm.

[26] http://www.fda.gov/regulatoryinformation/guidances/ucm125067.htm.

[27] http://www.accessdata.fda.gov/scripts/cdrh/cfdocs/cfCFR/CFRSearch.cfm?CFRPart=1
      1&showFR=1.

[28] Foldit game. http://en.wikipedia.org/wiki/Foldit; Accessed 5/26/2013.

[29] Infosys.com.

[30] Davis S, Palmer M. The true cost of your prescription drugs. US Department of Com-
      merce. http://rense.com/general54/preco.htm; Accessed 5/2/2013.

[31] Gonce A, Schrader U. Plantopia? A mandate for innovation in pharma manufacturing.
      McKinsey & Co.

[32] Biswas K. Pharma Gain from Information. SETLabs Briefings. May 2008.

[33] Millipore. Mobius® CellReady Single-use Bioreactor Systems. http://www.millipore.
      com/techpublications/tech1/ds3377en00; Accessed 5/21/2013.

[34] http://www.pharmacy.ca.gov/about/e_pedigree_laws.shtml.

[35] Implanted blood monitor can signal heart attack via smartphone. http://www.washing-
      tontimes.com/news/2013/mar/24/implanted-blood-monitor-can-signal-heart-attack-
      sm/; Accessed 5/26/2013.

[36] Adherence. http://obssr.od.nih.gov/scientific_areas/health_behaviour/adherence/index.a
      spx; Accessed 4/28/2013.

[37]–[40] Biswas K. Emerging Markets: The Time is Right to Invest. Pharma September/October
           2011.

[41] Biswas K. Cut Your IT Costs With Shared Services. http://www.pharmexec.com/pharm
      exec/author/authorInfo.jsp?id=53167.

Index

Note: Page numbers followed by "*f*" denote figures; "*t*" tables.

www.ingramcontent.com/pod-product-compliance
Lightning Source LLC
Chambersburg PA
CBHW060554220326
41598CB00024B/3099